ORGASMS THAT WILL MAKE HER TOES CURL

ORGASMS
THAT WILL MAKE
HER TOES CURL

THE MANY AMAZING WAYS TO CLIMAX—AS ONLY A WOMAN CAN

LISA SWEET

Amorata Press

Published by: AMORATA PRESS,
               an imprint of Ulysses Press
               P.O. Box 3440
               Berkeley, CA 94703
               www.amoratapress.com

ISBN13: 978-1-56975-870-0
Library of Congress Control Number: 2010915353

Printed in the United States by Bang Printing

10 9 8 7 6 5 4 3 2 1

Acquisitions editor: Keith Riegert
Managing editor: Claire Chun
Copyeditors: Mark Rhynsburger, Lauren Harrison
Proofreader: Lily Chou
Design and layout: Wade Nights
Production: Abigail Reser, Judith Metzener
Photographs: © Hollan Publishing, Inc.

Distributed by Publishers Group West

Contents

Introduction	7
1 X Marks the Spot	11
2 Going Sol-Oh!	43
3 Getting Handy	67
4 Mouthing Off	83
5 All the Right Moves	105
6 Advanced Techniques	137

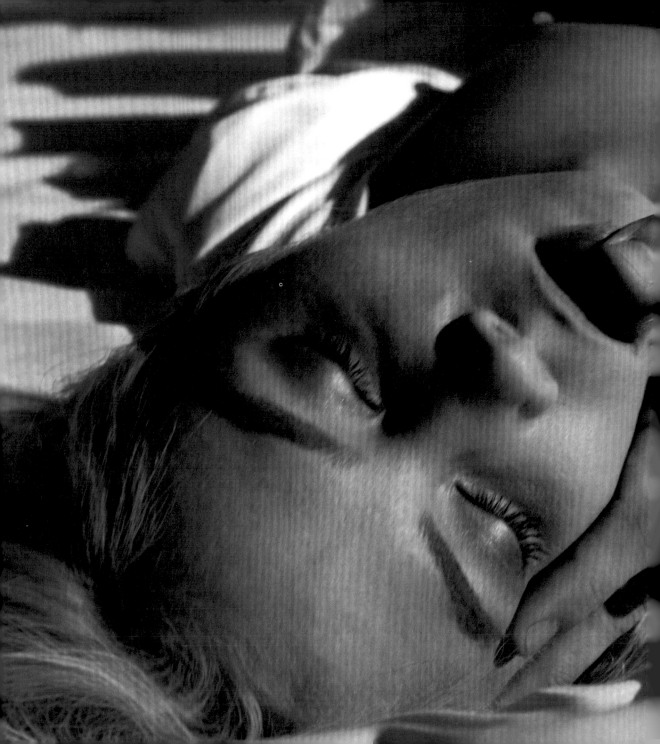

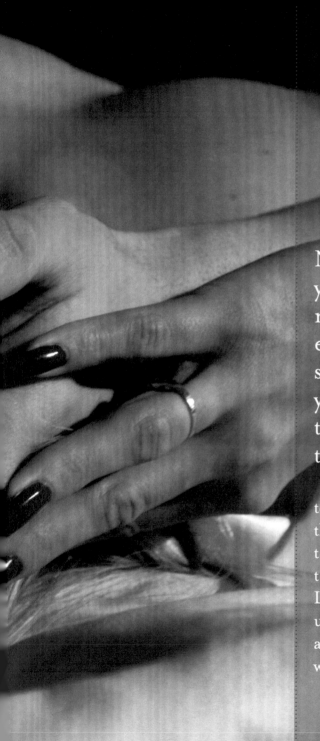

Orgasms That Will Make Her Toes Curl

No matter how much you love your sex life, it can always be made a bit more joyful. So even though you have your signature move that pushes your orgasm buttons every time, that doesn't mean it's the only way.

From mini concentrated jolts of bliss to deep, full-body feel-good explosions, this book is full of mattress-tested tips, techniques, and triggers guaranteed to make you very, very happy in bed. Luckily, it doesn't take much for you to unlock your enormous sexual potential and experience moments of delight whenever and as often as you desire.

Yes, Yes, Yes, Seven Times Yes!

Having an orgasm isn't like playing a va-va-voom lottery. There are quite a few things a woman can do to put herself on the inside fast track to nirvana. All are so easy you'll only sweat if you want to.

3.

Ignore your V zone—stretching out foreplay intensifies the final shebang. By paying homage to your other la-di-da spots, he stokes your fires until *whoosh!* Called *peaking*, this simple sexual technique not only increases the release of endorphins, it also teaches your body to stay in a practically permanent orgasmic pleasure zone so you're able to keep on partying.

2.

Break a sweat. Any activity that raises the heart rate—like a brisk walk, bike ride, or 15 minutes on the treadmill—is a perfect passion primer. Exercise equals endorphins—the all-natural chemicals produced by the body to get a person all hot under the collar. Are your sweats not exactly your seduce-me-now outfit? Just crank some get-down-with-it tunes and shimmy. Make it aerobic by throwing in some lap dance bumps and grinds.

1.

The best sex starts long before a couple gets down and dirty. One surefire way to get into a steamy state of mind is for you to put "hot thoughts" on your daily task list. Get him in on your steamy act by leaving a provocative sticky note for him or sending a suggestive text midday.

4.

Know how to occasionally throw his emergency brake. Most guys take between 2 and 10 minutes to go limp with joy—whereas you'll take around 20. Do the math. The solution is for you both to back off and focus on you when he seems to be approaching the point of no return. One tip to help him last longer: Have him penetrate as usual, but when he feels like he's about to pull the trigger, move his hips in a circular motion (like swaying a hula hoop) until things calm down.

5.

Just as the penis has a shaft, the clitoris has a layer of tissue called a hood that, like a piece of high-performance fabric, is thick enough to protect the nerves from overstimulation yet thin enough to allow a build-up of pleasurable friction. With all that engineering, he can rub you into a frenzy.

6.

Spread your joy. You've got a better chance of having more than one orgasm if he shifts his moves around—for example, switching from oral to intercourse, to using his fingers, to stimulating your G-spot.

7.

Realize that there is never such a thing as too much clitoris. Little known fact: the little nub of flesh is only the tip of a complex system of nerve endings that lead back into your body and down your inner thighs.

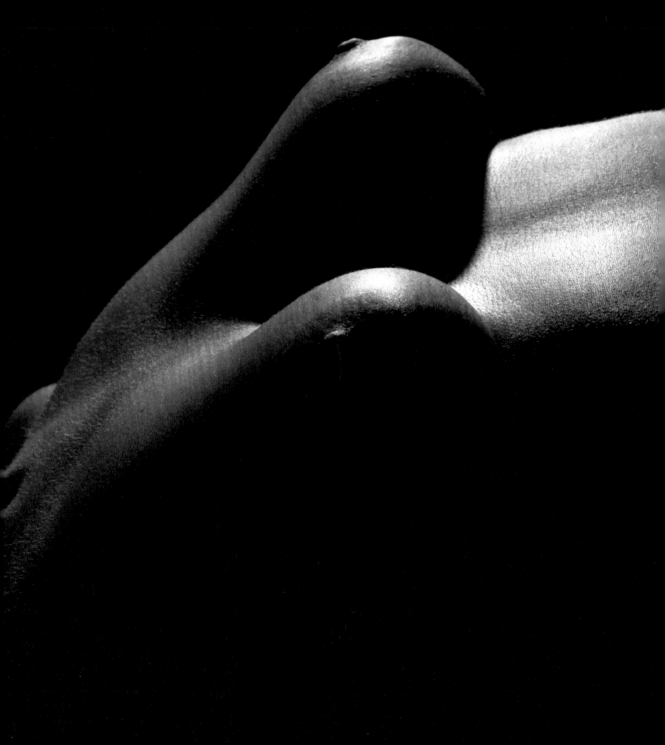

1: X MARKS THE SPOT

Women are especially primed to feel good in oh! so many ways, but you probably don't realize how adaptable your body is. All it takes is the merest touch to one of your many nerve-packed, spine-tingling erogenous zones to take you from 0 to…69 in seconds.

True, each person has her own special areas, but there are some fail-safe spots located around the entire body that are guaranteed to please. Knees? Neck? Behind ears? What turns you on? Packed with thrill power, these happy buttons are capable of producing insane euphoria. Here's how to spot your orgasm.

Hot Spot Number 1: Mind Games

The mind is the epicenter of sex. Nothing happens anywhere else until this zone is primed and primped for some hanky-panky. It doesn't matter how great his technique is. If the organ between your ears isn't stimulated, your genitals won't lubricate, your sensations will become dulled, and sex will be blah.

GPS to Your Mind

Luckily, it doesn't take much to melt your mind since everything has the potential to be sexy. When he grabs your hand as you walk down the street, when he checks in with you in the middle of the day to tell you he's thinking of you, when he gives you his crooked grin—these are the things that make you mentally involved with a man.

On-the-Spot Bliss

Get ready to whimper with these frolic-maxing mental moves:

Concoct your own carnal code   Use something like the peace sign or finger-tugging an earlobe as a signal to your lover. This way, you can be at a party and flash your sexy signal to let each other know that maybe it's time to slip out—or just off to the bathroom for a quickie.

Get wordy   Even a little X-rated talk and frothy fantasies are guaranteed to heat things up. You can create an erotic story together. If you're shy, text it back and forth during the day. Work with open-ended primal phrases like "Three things I want you to do to me…" or "He moved his fingers over her…" or "She told him to…" A more hard-core move includes making up a fervid fantasy where he tells you exactly how he intends to have his wicked, wontan way with you later.

Get daydreamy   All it takes is a few extra seconds to turn your day into one long erotic fest. Start by sensuously rubbing on your body lotion in the morning. When you rummage through the closet, slip into clothes that make you feel like Miss Thing, even if it's just some leggings that show off your booty. Last, take a few minutes during the day to have a sex break. No touching necessary—simply think about the caresses that make you pant.

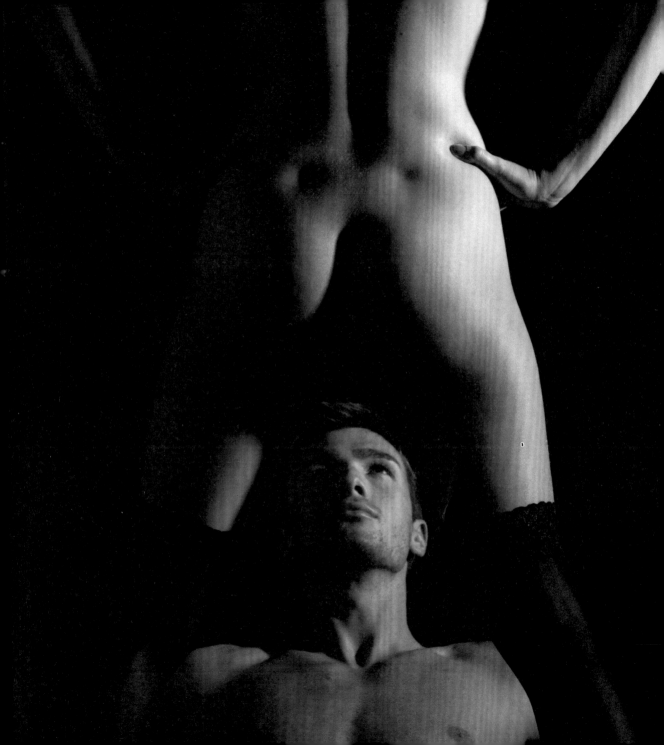

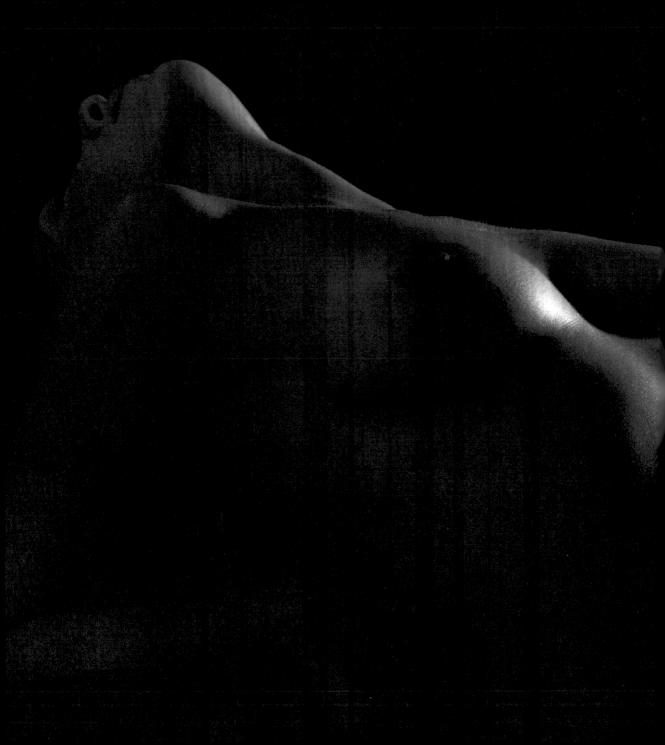

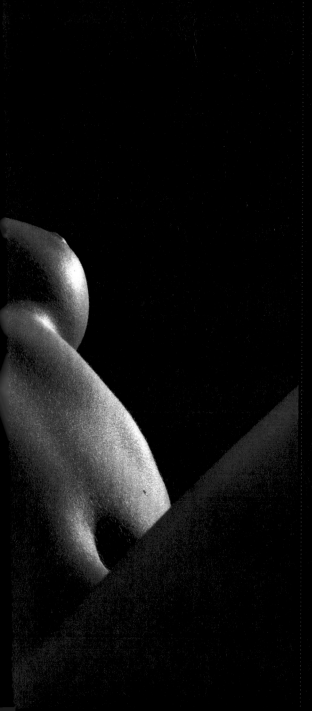

Hot Spot Number 2: The Skin

The largest hot spot is the skin—which means there's oh! so much more to enjoy beyond the small diamond between your legs. The skin is literally packed with nerves that respond to different temperatures, pressures, and strokes. Multiply these by a person's individual tastes and desires, and the routes to arousal seem endless.

GPS to Your Skin

Every inch of your body (and his) is a hotbed of sensual potential, but the cream-of-the-crop spots are where the skin is very thin. Nerves are closer to the surface here, making it more responsive to stimulation. The best way to set your desire on fire is not just to stroke these areas, but to use caresses that parallel the nerve pathways so every inch of skin is stirred.

On-the-Spot Bliss

A connect-the-dots guide for him in how to lick, squeeze, and stroke you into orgasmic overdrive:

Mouth corners   Licking around these edges will put you on the erotic edge.

Ears   Swirling a tongue gently along the outer rim will set off an amazing chain reaction of rapture.

Front of neck   Because it's off the beaten passion path, this area doesn't get much amorous

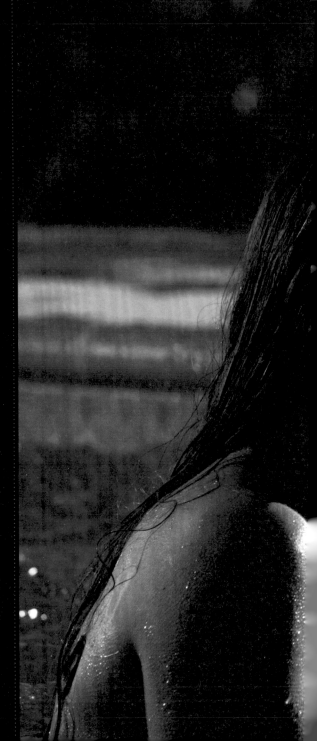

attention. But caressing here will cause goose bumps all over. Lie back so your neck is arched forward, making it easy for him to lap long, lazy licks straight up and down from just below your chin to the small hollow where your rib cage starts.

Face When he places two fingers on each temple and gently presses at the same time, the stress will let loose and pure pleasure will take over.

Inner arms Swooping sweeps from elbow to wrist will really rouse you, particularly if he uses a feather.

Palms A few soft, ever-expanding strokes of this patch of skin can add an erotic punch to holding hands. Using his fingertips to trace widening circles from the center to the entire palm may even set off a hands-on orgasm.

Mons Keeping to the unexplored patch above the genitals where the pubic hair grows can be so scorching it'll set your desire on fire—especially if his next stop is what lies below.

Back The whole spine shivers to the touch but the lower part, just above the buttocks, is gasp central. Running a tongue along the length of your backbone before settling in for some nuzzling there will make you want to sit up straight, especially if he ups the erotic ante by sucking on an ice cube before he begins.

Inner thighs Alternating between licking and gently nibbling in teeny-tiny circles will make you want to twist and shout.

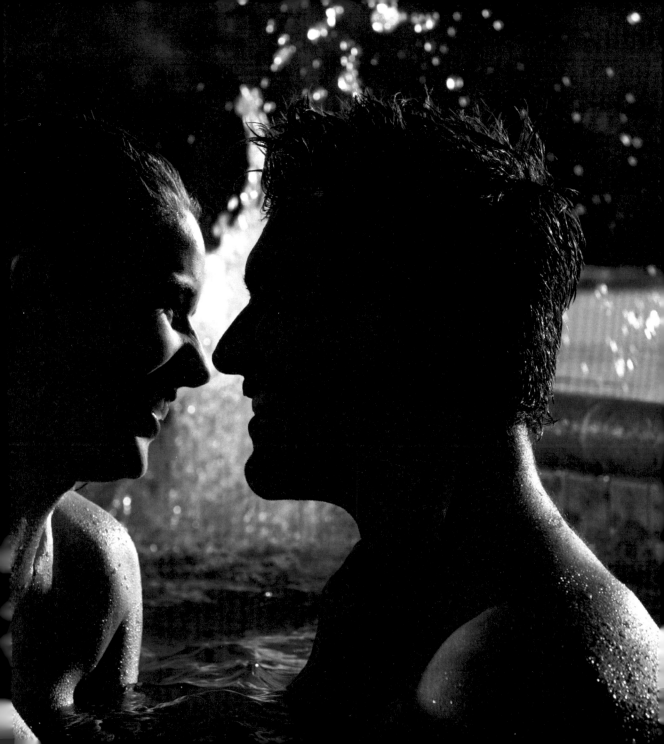

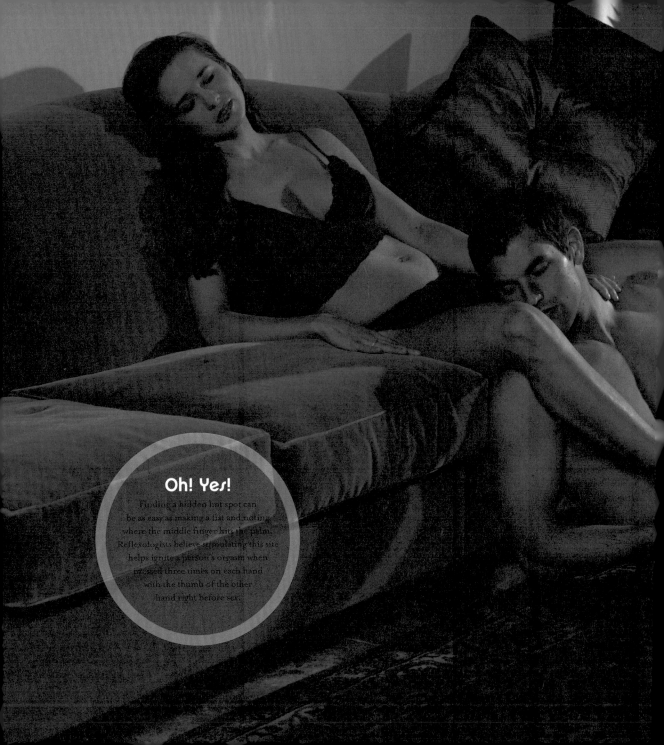

Oh! Yes!

Finding a hidden hot spot can
be as easy as making a fist and noting
where the middle finger hits the palm.
Reflexologists believe stimulating this site
helps ignite a person's orgasm when
pressed three times on each hand
with the thumb of the other
hand right before sex.

Oh! No!

Hot-spot hunting will turn ice cold if you aren't already hot and sticky. This means your clitoris is erect, your entire labial and urethral sponge areas are swollen, and you are very, very wet. If these conditions don't exist, he'll only succeed in irritating you— not exactly the happy ending you were hoping for.

Back of the knees Off-the-beaten path, crisscrossing strokes that start here and gradually sweep from your ankles to your bottom will make you want to roll over and beg for mercy.

Foot rub There are trigger points in the feet that, when touched, cause an electric current to buzz straight up between your legs. (According to reflexology, there are nearly 7,000 nerves in your dogs.) Massage some lotion with both hands in a circular motion from the center of each foot outward to the heel and toes: This will knead you into a happy haze.

Head-to-toe touch Being sudsed up by your partner in the shower will awaken your entire body, especially if he soaps himself up first and then wraps you in a slippery, sliding embrace under a cascade of lukewarm water.

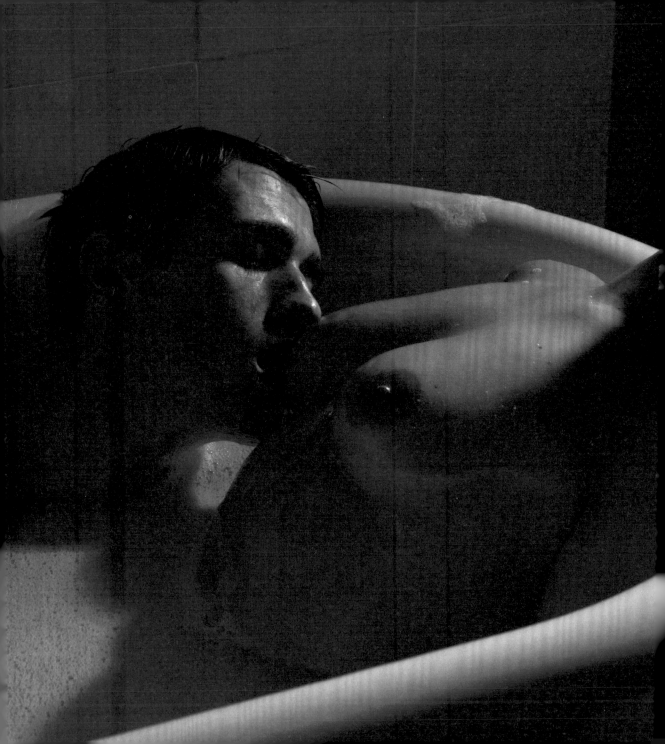

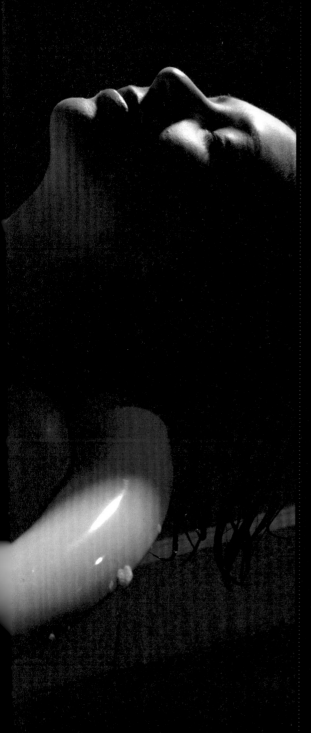

Hot Spot Number 3: Best Breasts

You know that your nipples are your bliss blossoms. But the entire breast area is rich in tender spots, and while the bliss quotient doesn't vary with the size of the cup, the type of caress does.

GPS to Your Breasts

You certainly know how to find your breasts and nipples, and he (hopefully) does, too. But you may not know that the areola, the darker-skinned area that surrounds the nipple, also responds to a little tender loving care, as do the breasts' fleshy outer areas.

On-the-Spot Bliss

The areola is actually paradise central, no matter what size your breasts. The top part of the areola—"north" of the nipple—especially makes you raring to go when caressed in soft full circles. He can up the pressure with kisses that create a constant sensation of suction.

Touch   Featherlight spiral moves over the entire area will keep you from feeling any uncomfortable friction. But once the action gets going, he can pinch, flick, squeeze, and jiggle to his heart's delight—and yours.

Double up   He can slide his penis between your orbs while slipping his tongue between your legs.

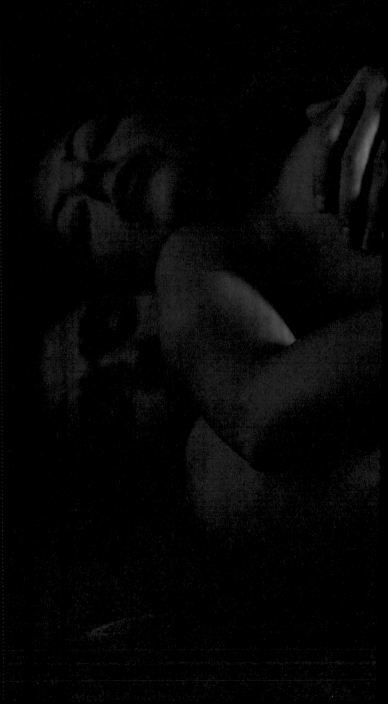

Hot Spot Number 4: The Big C

You know where your clitoris is and what it's capable of—now you need to make sure he does, too! Bottom line: The clitoris has over 8,000 nerve fibers, more than there are inside the vagina. That's a lot of sensitivity right there, which is why it's easier for many women to orgasm when there's some clitoral action thrown into play.

But while a clitoris may be similar to a penis, it's not a penis. It doesn't respond to the kind of firm pressure that leaves him gasping. If even the lightest touch can shower you with sonic sensations, imagine how painful a rough, careless touch can be. Which is why he needs to keep it light—that is, until you beg for more.

GPS to Your Clitoris

You probably think your clitoris is just a small, hard-to-find nugget between your outer lips. But that's just the tip of the iceberg. The

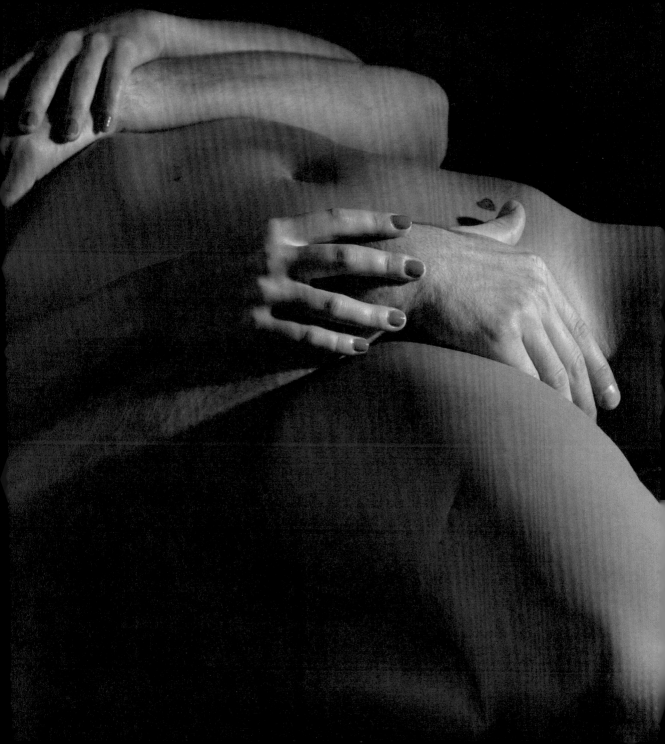

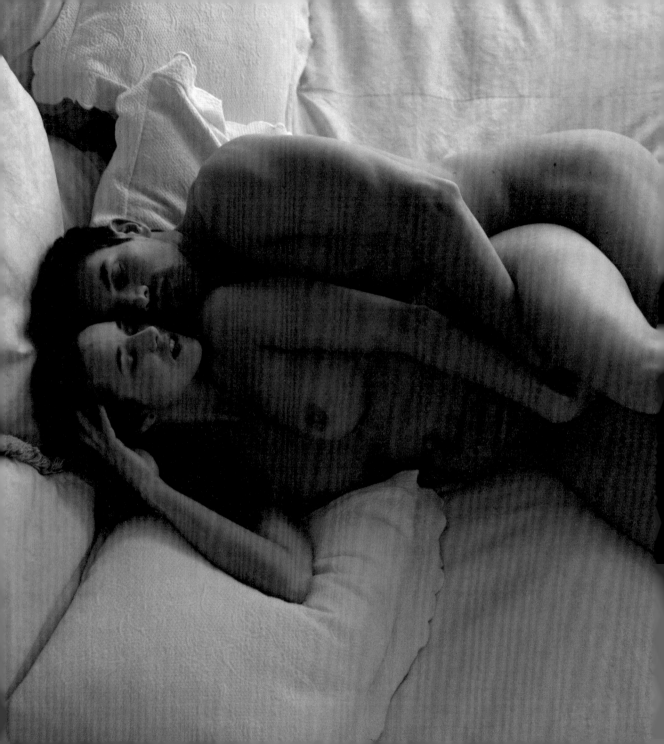

Oh! No!

Pressing a dry clitoris will have the same effect as rubbing sandpaper all over your skin. If you aren't producing your own juices, you can keep things moist with some over-the-counter lube (make sure it's compatible with your birth control) or a few drops of spit.

Oh! Yes!

One half of your clitoris is often more sensitive—and quicker to bring pleasure—than the other. To feel which side he can use to put you into hyperdrive, bend one leg at the knee and angle it out while straightening the other leg so it's in line with your body. Then switch.

part you don't see, which is buried inside and runs along the lower pubic bones, forks out into two long, separate legs. The overall length of the clitoris, measured inside and out, is about four inches—close to the length of an unerect penis. (Yes, four inches— no matter what he says!) So if you're amazed that something so tiny can be so incredibly sensitive don't be. It's not so tiny after all. When stimulated in the right way this inner clitoris can set off melt- down orgasms.

On-the-Spot Bliss

To get a sense of the lay of the land he can form a *V* with his index and middle fingers and point them toward your feet. Pressing this *V* so that a finger is to each side of the clitoris will zero in on your love button, especially if he pulls up slightly.

To get a feel for what's going on inside, he can push down on your lower abdomen with outstretched fingers, massaging the skin on either side of your vagina in a scissors motion, causing the skin of your inner labia to caress the shaft

Oh! Yes!

Don't freak—that liquid spurting out of you probably isn't pee. Some women experience such an exquisite ecstasy when they have a G-spot orgasm that they actually ejaculate a clear, silky fluid through their urethra.

Oh! No!

Because the G-spot is so close to the urethra, touching it may trigger that urgent gotta-go feeling, as if you have to urinate. The problem? You clench up and don't let go, so no climax. Try peeing before sex so you can relax when the moment comes.

Hot Spot Number 5:
Gee Whiz

In the front wall of your vagina lives a soft swelling called the G-spot that will make you scream with joy when it's pressed. G-spot (aka Grafenberg spot) orgasms are intense, whole-body sexperiences that have been known to produce the surprising and amazing effect of female ejaculation.

GPS to Your G-Spot

The G-spot is an ultrasensitive mass of tissue roughly a third of the way up the front wall of the vagina. It feels like a soft marshmallow when touched. The easiest way for him to find it: Have him hold his palm face up and gently slip a well-lubed finger or two inside your vagina, then curl them into a "come hither" position and softly feel along the front wall. The G-spot will feel rougher than the surrounding area and slightly ridged.

It helps if attention is also given your nipples, clitoris, and anything else that gets your motor running. The more revved you are, the more your G will stand out, making it easier to locate. If you feel a slight urge to urinate when it gets pressed, don't worry.

This sensation should soon give way to intensifying delight.

On-the-Spot Bliss

Once he's on location, these simple sleights of hand will work some G-spot magic.

1. Rhythm is everything—he should keep his diddling slow, steady, and sturdy.

2. He can use his thumb to give you a G-spot jiggy. After slipping his index and middle fingers inside and pressing against your G, he curls around with his thumb to say hello to your clitoris.

3. Once he's hit the spot, ask him to massage it in slow, gentle circles.

4. The G can take a lot of pressure, so you may want to ask him to press harder.

5. Get him to tap dance, striking firmly and repeatedly on your G-spot. This constant pressure will build waves of sensation, finishing in an incredible climax.

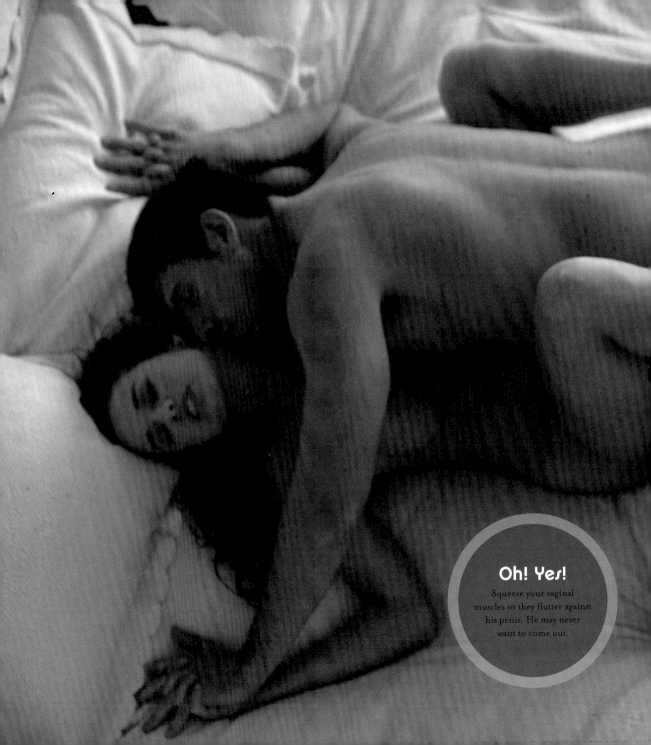

Oh! Yes!

Squeeze your vaginal
muscles so they flutter against
his penis. He may never
want to come out.

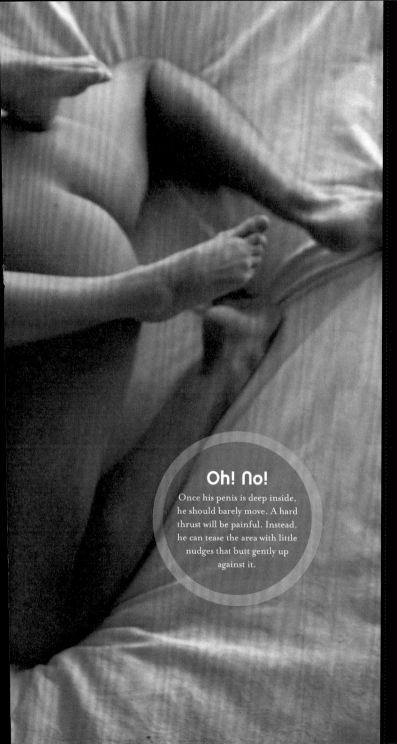

Hot Spot Number 6: Hit a High C

The cervix is the tubelike out-cropping of hard tissue at the back of your vagina that acts as a gateway to your uterus. Highly sensitive, it can create an OMG feeling when pressed.

GPS to Your Cervix

This is a no-hands-required hot spot. His penis is made just right to give your cervix all the loving it needs.

On-the-Spot Bliss

Train his penis to tango with your cervix:

- He needs to penetrate fully, but, once he's in, he should mix up his usual in-and-out moves with a few circular rotations and figure eights.

- He can withdraw just a bit before diving in deep again so he's almost tapping against your cervix with his tip.

Oh! No!

Once his penis is deep inside, he should barely move. A hard thrust will be painful. Instead, he can tease the area with little nudges that butt gently up against it.

Hot Spot Number 7: Ahhhh Zone

The anterior fornix erogenous zone, also known as the AFE zone or A-spot, is a vortex of nerves that carries information from your whole genital region to the spinal cord and brain. When stimulated, these nerves send hot-and-heavy signals to the part of your nervous system that juices up your libido. When pressed just so, many women report having the most intense orgasm of their lives.

GPS to Your AFE

The AFE is located on the front wall of the vagina, a third of the way down from the cervix. To find it, slide moistened fingers up your vagina until you hit your G-spot. If he's getting in on the action, he can stop and play for a while before continuing on up the wall to the cervix at the back of the vaginal canal. Once there, he backs down until he's midway between your cervix and your G-spot. It'll feel smooth and extremely sensitive to the touch. That's the AFE.

He'll know he's in the right place if he presses and is knocked back by waves of muscular contractions that seem hell-bent on pushing him right out of you. When this happens, get him to push back. The more he pushes into you forcefully, the more powerful your ultimate pleasure payoff will be.

On-the-Spot Bliss

A couple of pressing moves to make you cry "A-ha!"

- He can slide a finger up and down, using the G-spot and cervix as his boundaries. Right in between these two, he'll find this pleasure pocket.

- He can use two fingers to stroke the AFE zone and then lightly rub the sides of the walls—first clockwise halfway and then counterclockwise halfway.

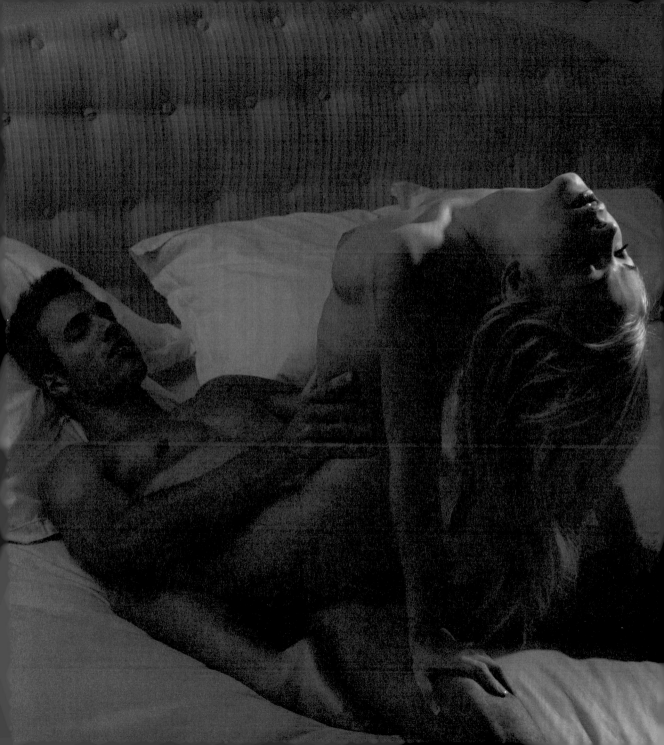

Oh! Yes!
A dab of lube maximizes his chances of stimulating rather than irritating your urethra.

Oh! No!
The urethral area is infection-prone, so hands should be well scrubbed before heading over to it.

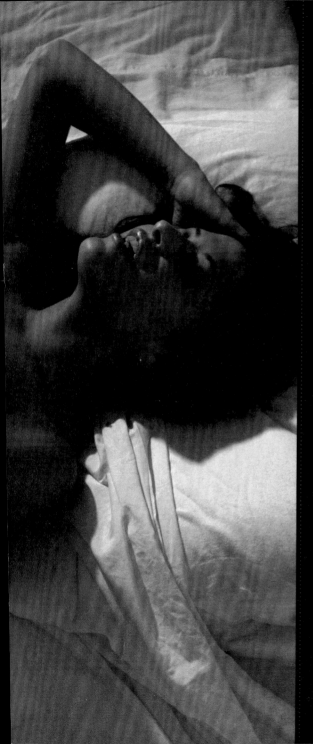

Hot Spot Number 8: U-Reka!

The area surrounding the urethral opening is supersensitive. During sex, it begins to enlarge and swell. When delicately stimulated, it creates a soft, melting kind of climax.

GPS to Your Urethra

The urethra is the tiny area of tissue below the clitoris that includes the opening that you pee from. The joy comes not from the actual opening but just above and to either side of it. As with the G-spot, if the urethra is pressed just so, you may actually ejaculate.

On-the-Spot Bliss

✦ Using one or two fingers, he can alternate between the following motions or just stick with one: a gentle but firm sliding up-and-down stroke or a continual circular motion.

✦ If he's on the fast track to orgasm, he can speed you up by focusing on your clitoris with his tongue but using his lower lip (bracing it against his teeth to avoid nips) to apply strong, constant pressure to your urethra.

✦ The urethra is a great place to shift his mouth after you've had an orgasm and your clitoris is feeling too sensitive for direct stimulation.

Hot Jpot Number 9: Pleasure Booty

Your bottom and perineum are often-missed hot spots, but these areas are crammed with sensitive nerves guaranteed to raise your orgasmic quotient. No anal sex required.

GPJ to Your Butt

The perineum is also sometimes called the "taint." This comes from an old joke: "It ain't the anus and it ain't the vagina." But it is worth finding.

Both men and women have this spine-tingling area. Composed of tissue similar to the vaginal lips and penis head, the perineum is chock-a-block with touchy-feely nerve endings that start humming when aroused. If you've ever had your toes curl from riding a horse, bike, or motorcycle, it's probably because you piqued your perineum. To locate yours, think of your lower region as a diamond with the vaginal opening at the center. The perineum is the southernmost point of this shape. It is the little stretch of flesh between the anal and vaginal openings.

Then there are the buns, of course. But the anal opening is also brimming with throbbing nerve tips that tingle to the touch.

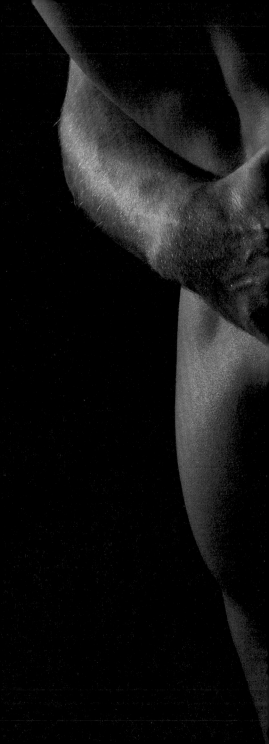

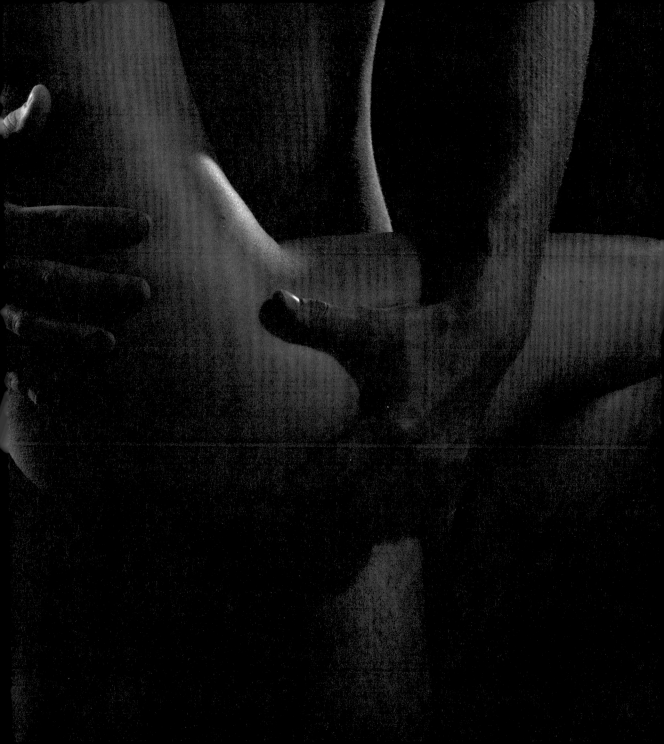

On-the-Spot Bliss

An easy-to-please all-purpose hot zone that's easy to fire up.

❖ Due to the perineum's prime position between the anal and vaginal openings, he can stroke all three areas, keeping you guessing where the next good feeling is coming from.

❖ The P-zone is a good place for him to take a rest stop when doing oral laps around your clitoris because it can be bitten, sucked, or licked.

❖ Massaging the perineum can help the pelvic muscles relax, which increases blood flow and makes both vaginal and anal penetration easier.

❖ He can squeeze, pinch, knead, and even lightly slap your bottom, or he can slip one clean, well-lubed finger up into your backdoor and see what comes.

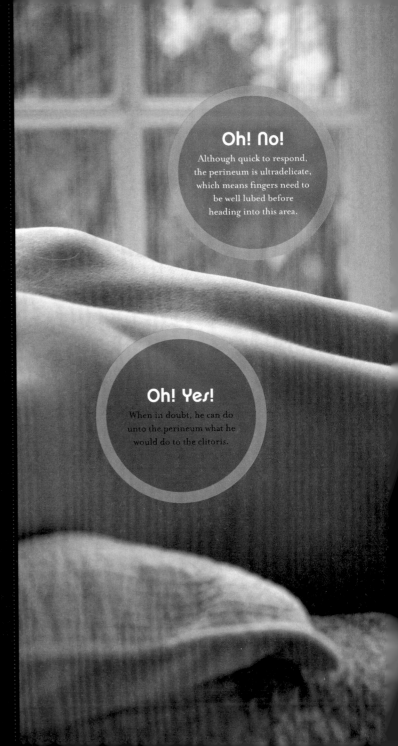

Oh! No!

Although quick to respond, the perineum is ultradelicate, which means fingers need to be well lubed before heading into this area.

Oh! Yes!

When in doubt, he can do unto the perineum what he would do to the clitoris.

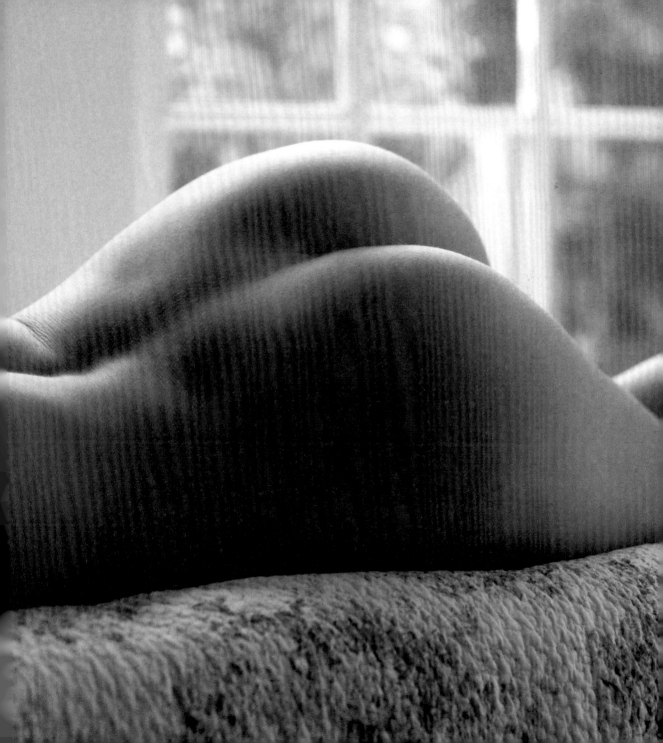

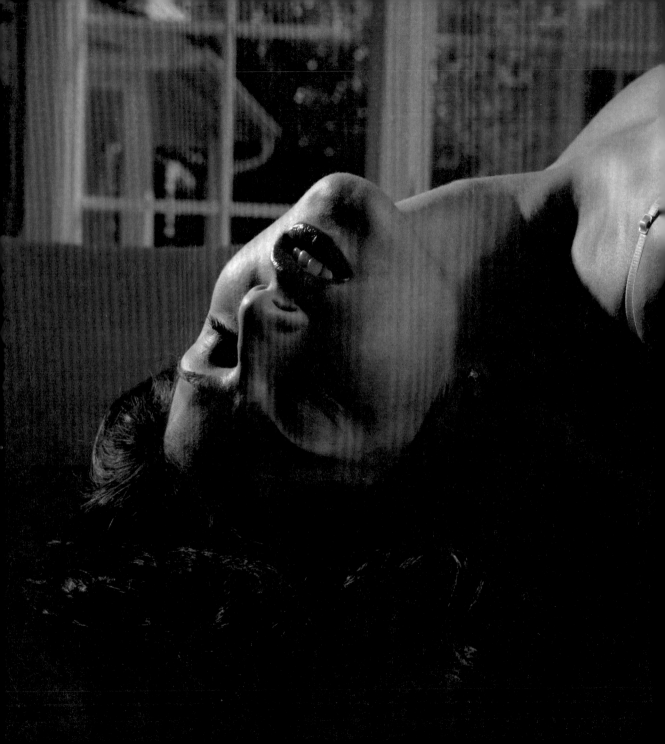

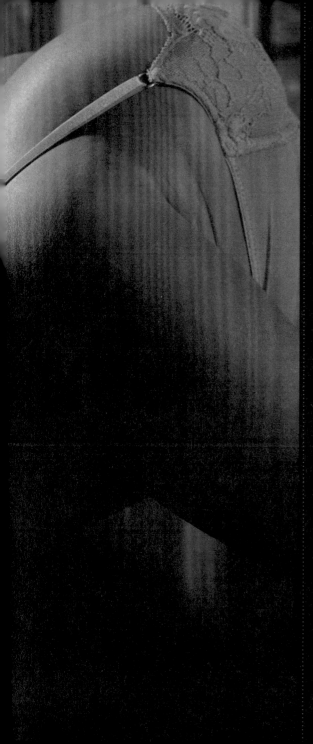

Blended Bliss

Women have two paths to nirvana—vaginal and clitoral. But, lucky girl, you don't have to settle for just one kind of bliss. Maximum joy is at hand when he can caress all three parts of what's called the orgasmic crescent—a curved area that extends from your clitoral tip across your urethral opening, into your vagina, past your G-spot, and up to your AFE zone.

◈ To blitz all your bits at once, he can use all of his newly honed skills to manually or orally touch both the clitoral tip and the U-spot while simultaneously applying pressure to the G-spot. If you're up for it, he can slide up to your AFE zone.

◈ If you want to try a big bang during intercourse, get on top so his penis slants to hit your G-spot. As you're riding happy, he grabs your hips and massages your clitoris with his thumbs. If you can keep your balance after that, push down hard so he presses against your cervix.

◈ Finally, for the truly flexible, lie on your back and raise your legs. Your partner can grab an ankle in each hand and literally maneuver your limbs closed or wide open, or one forward and the other back, to create some superintense, knee-buckling, below-the-belt action.

On-the-Spot Bliss for Him

Take a joy trip to his hot spots. Like you, your man has plenty of Big O buttons, too. Here are the ABCs to finding his moan zones.

Fondle his F-spot   The frenulum is the vertical ridge that extends along the underside of the penis from the tip to the shaft. Stroking it will hit his climax switch. Not only are there more nerve endings there, but the skin is also extremely thin.

Best move   Clenching your pelvic muscles just as he pulls out will give his F-spot a massage.

Rub his R-spot   Many men are surprised to discover the range and depth of the sensation when you caress their raphe, the visible line down the middle of the scrotum, between the testicles. He may even end up ejaculating sooner than he (and you) planned.

Best move   Excite the raphe by gently running your fingertips along it.

Press His P-spot   A man's erection doesn't end at the base of the penis. There's a railroad junction full of nerves in the perineum, that smooth triangle of flesh between the base of his penis and his anus, which, when pressed, will send him straight into an orgasmic swoon.

Best move   Gently rub the spot with the pad of your finger or thumb. (Pressing really hard with one forceful push can actually stop him from peaking, so be careful.)

Gyrate his G-spot   Owing to the location of the prostate gland at the base of the penis, a man's erection is more or less anchored on the prostate—also known as the male G-spot.

Best move   Slip a well-lubricated finger through the rectum and probe the rectum's upper wall. When you feel a firm, rounded, walnut-size lump, gently caress while stroking his penis at the same time.

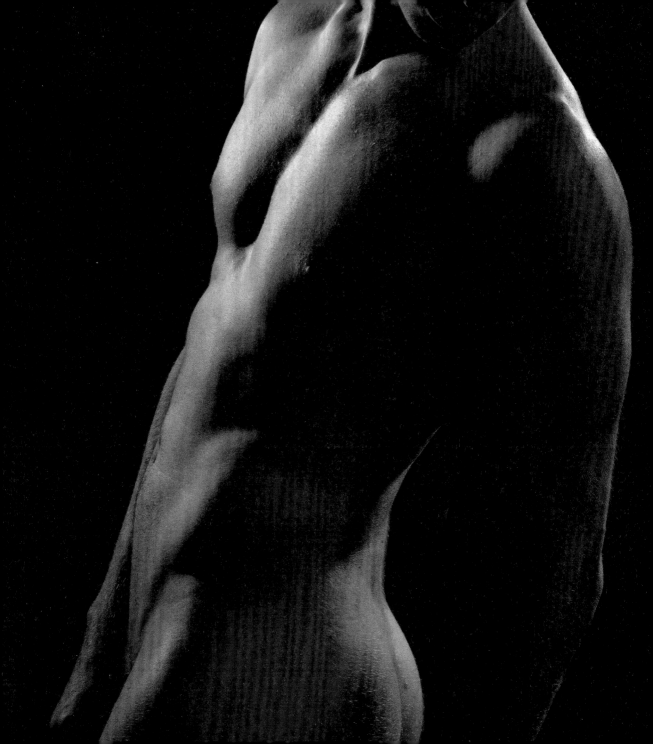

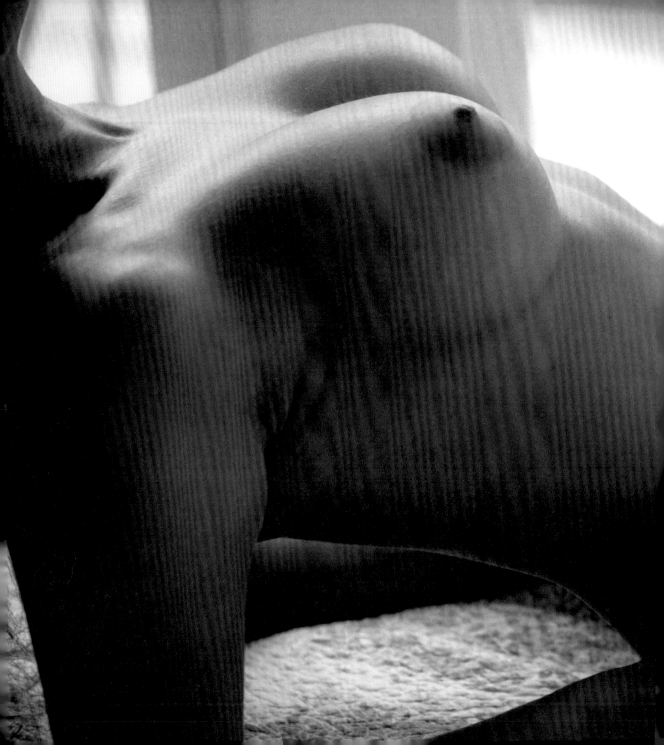

2: GOING SOL-OH!

Masturbation is, hands down, the surest path to orgasm: Most men and women can bring themselves to ecstasy within four minutes flat. (The fastest female runner can't even bust a mile that quickly—current record: 4:12:56.) That's less time than it takes to figure out which way the condom unrolls!

People tend to stick with what they know works. But this doesn't mean that your basic technique couldn't use a helping hand. A few new handy tricks could be all it takes to put an extra-goofy smile on your face.

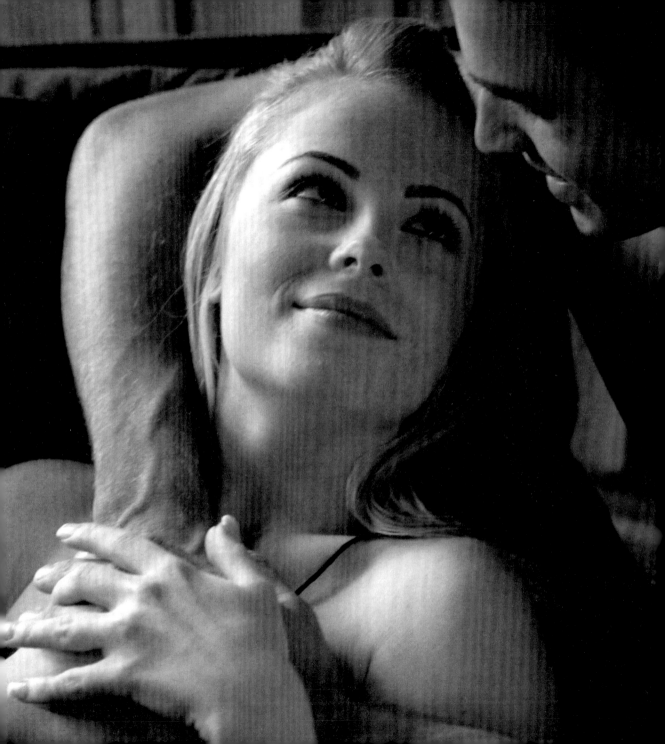

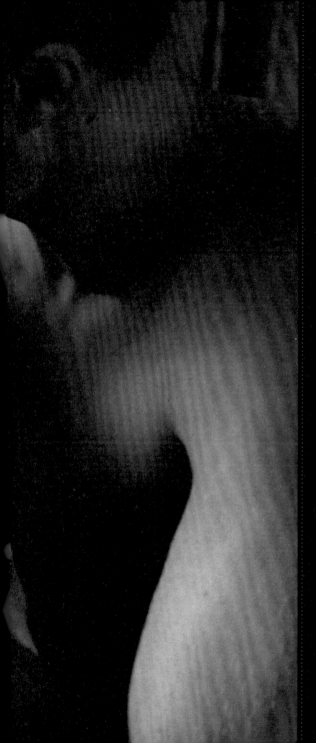

But using the same routine over and over—no matter how yowza that method may be—can limit your (endless) erotic potential. First, there's no guarantee that your self-love MO is going to translate to love à deux. Also, eventually, on-the-side-using-two-hands will start feeling as stale as last year's fashion must-have. Only this is what your body is now used to and has come to expect, so you're going to need to start from scratch to find out all the delightful ways you can make yourself feel good. There are worse assignments in life!

So it makes sense that the more ways you can hit your thrill switch, the more likely you are to feel that familiar ting-a-ling-ling no matter who you share your sheets with. Luckily, there are as many different ways to get yourself off as there are women masturbating.

It's not that this kind of exploration isn't possible with a partner. But if you're trying to figure out the mechanics of what feels good during sex, it would require patience, muscle control, communication, and staying power on his end. When you have the bed to yourself, you can make endless tiny adjustments—move your wrist slightly to the left, increase pressure, wiggle it back and forth—without having to direct him like a drill sergeant or worry about pulling his trigger prematurely. Then, when you're cuddling up with your honey, you can just get down to the business at hand: making each other feel fabulous.

Before You Touch

Make a love date with yourself   Every woman has her in-the-mood triggers when getting ready for sex. You can give yourself the same loving care even when you're preparing for a solo session—lighting candles, downloading a personal passion playlist, slipping into something silky and barely there or even a hot-to-trot thong and pair of thigh-high stockings, and rubbing your skin with oil. The higher you jack up your sexual energy, the more intense the end result.

Keep your panties on   It can be pleasurable torture to play with yourself over your underwear, teasing and stroking through the fabric. You're building the anticipation, so when you do end up going for skin-on-skin contact, it'll be that much more explosive and exciting.

Screw your head   Fantasies that get your fire burning are key to boosting desire. Plus, it's the most effective way to turn off the parts of the brain connected with anxiety and the never-ending to-do list. It doesn't matter who plays the starring role in your lusty daydreams—your partner, your boss, your neighbor. Some women are so mentally synched with their physical desires that they can actually think their way to climax. But there's plenty of female-friendly porn available online for those who need a nudge with the plot.

Don't pick a position   Make a habit of masturbating while assuming a variety of positions—lying on your back, on your stomach,

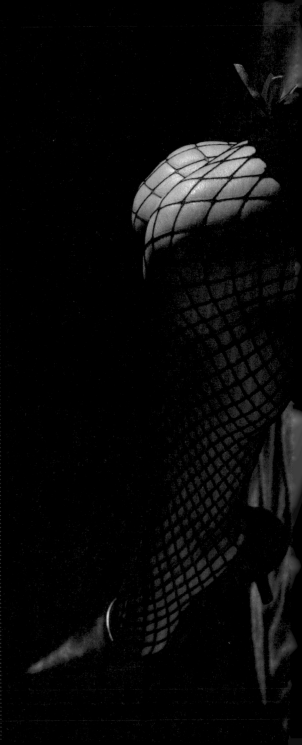

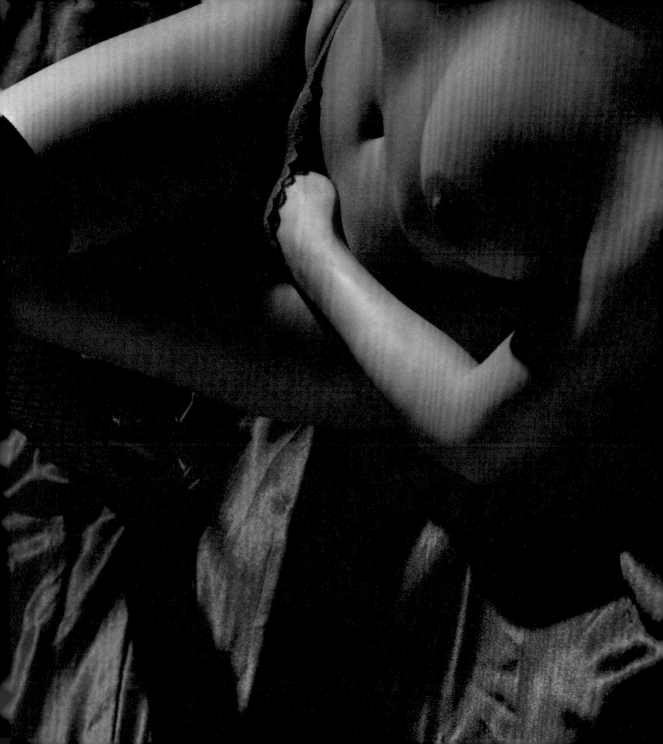

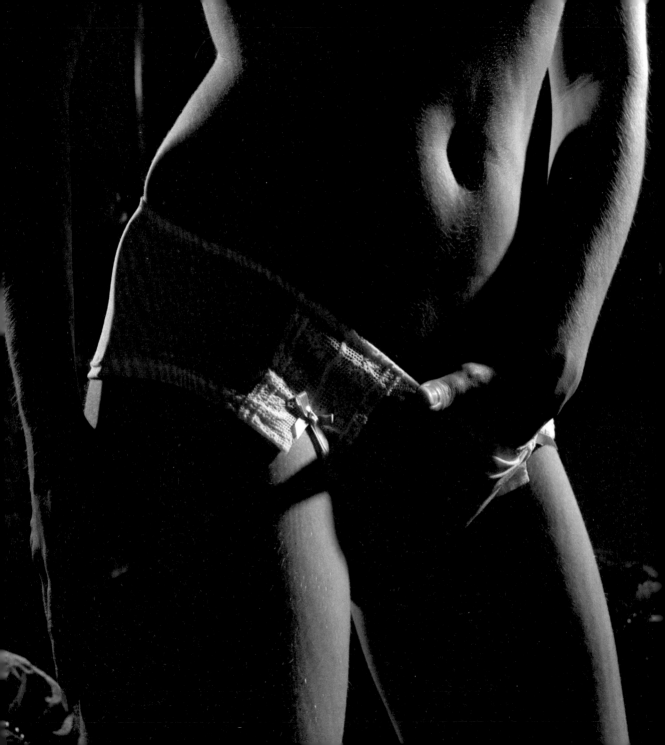

kneeling upright on the bed, bent over on hands and knees, cuddling up in a chair with your legs hooked over the sides. This lets you know your preferred stimulation in each pose for reaching your passion peak. You should always try a few rolls around the hay to test-drive different spots and see which works best today. Preferences change, depending on where you are in your cycle or how tired you feel or whether your tummy feels like a six-pack or a pack of pudge that day.

Grease up   Women have (rather handy) built-in lubrication systems, but that doesn't mean you might not need a few extra drops to juice things up, especially when you start. You can use a commercial lubricant or even a smidgeon of spit to moisten the action.

Pay attention   Even though you can make it happen fast, take your time and take mental notes on where you're touching, how much pressure you're applying, and what makes your toes clench. This will make it easier for you to re-create those same moves with your partner during sex.

Squeeze it   Simply squeezing or rubbing your thighs together can make the clitoris stand up and take notice. Bonus: This technique can even be used in public without risk, since you stay dressed so no one knows what you're up to. (In fact, the rub from your undies helps create extra friction.)

To become squeeze savvy, get into the habit of pressing your thighs together just as your body begins to melt down. Once this becomes second nature, jazz up the pressure: Continue to press your thighs together, and then pull your hands away—leaving it up to your legs to push you over the top. It may take a few tries before you get into orgasmic cruise control, but like anything, practice makes perfect. Take it to the next level by crossing your legs as you squeeze, boosting the rub factor.

No Hands Allowed

It takes dedicated DIY expertise to have an orgasm without touching yourself, but there is a Tantric method that the devoted can try to master. Called an "energy orgasm," it uses meditation to harness and direct one's *chi*, or life flow.

This isn't a speed-of-light affair, so here's an abbreviated version. (Still, allow yourself plenty of time.)

1. To begin, lie on a comfortable surface, flat on your back, arms at your sides with palms up. Inhale deeply though your nose and exhale through your mouth. This slow and steady way of breathing will help clear your mind and relax your body. Try not to let any pauses come between your breaths.

2. Once you've created a rhythm, begin to arch your lower back on the inhale and flatten it on the exhale. (Your pelvis will get into a rock-and-rolling rhythm.) Once you feel comfy, start squeezing your pubic muscles on the inhale as well. When you exhale, concentrate on letting your muscles relax. You'll know you have it right if it feels like your clitoris is being jazzed.

3. At the same time, try picturing a flow of energy entering your body through your toes. If you're on the right wavelength, you'll feel a tingle begin in your feet and move up your legs. As the tingle buzzes up your body, charge it with your breath as it passes through your chakras: groin, navel, heart, mouth, brow, and finally out through the top of your head.

4. Once you feel in control, focus on moving your breath between the chakras. This will be a bit tricky and take a number of tries before it feels easier. As you inhale and squeeze, imagine moving the energy in your body back and forth between your pubic muscles and the rest of your body via your breath.

5. If you're on the path to enlightenment, you'll feel an intense urge to touch yourself and even hold your breath. Resist! Continue to breathe deeply. With practice, you'll be able to power the intensity of your orgasm simply through your breath.

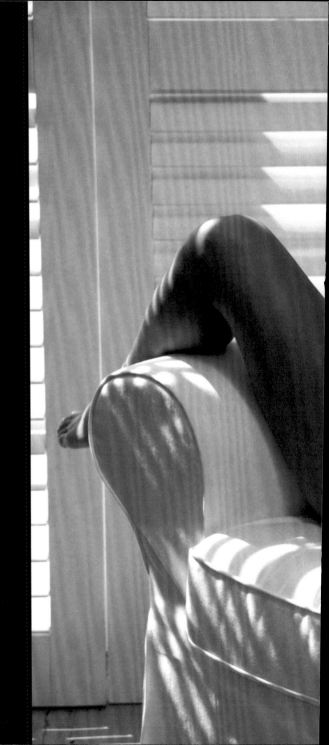

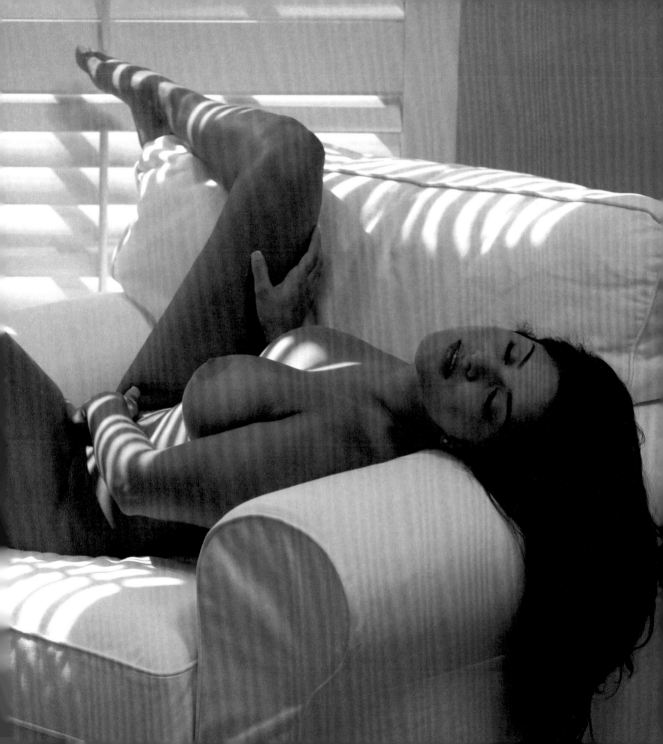

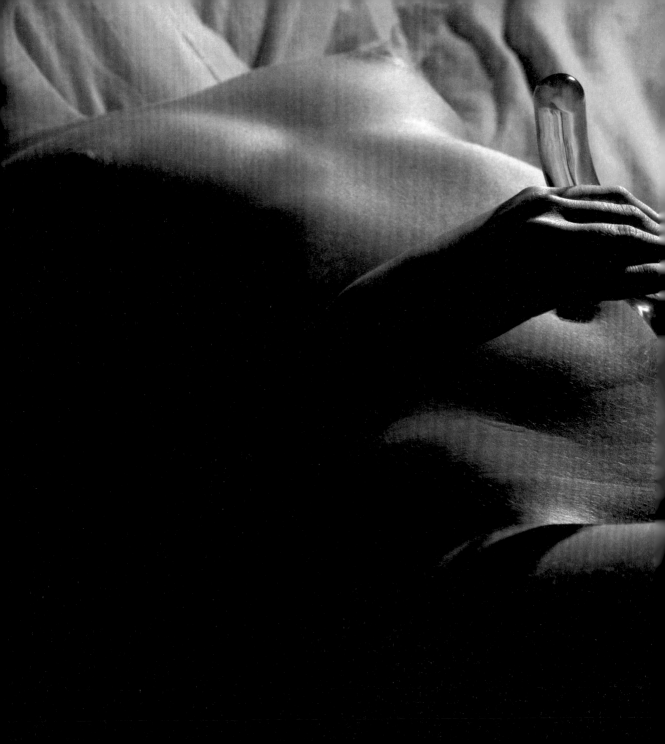

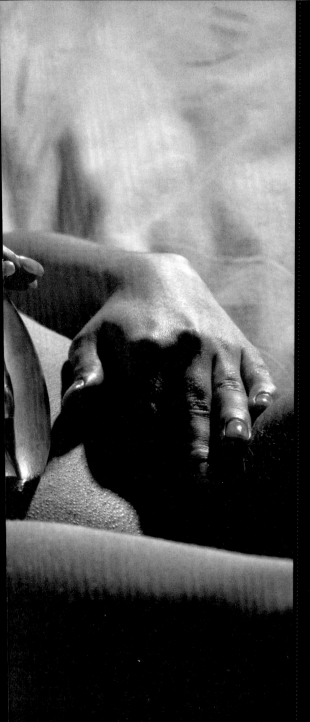

Exploring the Terrain

Most women don't mess around when it comes to taking their horny happiness into their own hands; they head straight for the gold and begin with their clitoris. But branch out and love up the rest of your body. Exploring it inside and out will help you discover your full orgasmic potential. Every inch of skin, from head to toes, is a potential source of glee—you never know which combination of touches will take you to your perky place. Though not as sensitive as that centrally located hot button, loads of other bits on your body are packed with layers of nerves that can produce unexpected sweet spots. A few fresh ways to get started:

✦ Many women have very sensitive breasts, and some can actually have a toe-curling moment from nipple stimulation alone. While you may not be that thin-skinned, giving the nips a squeeze, a tug, or a press when you're close to climax can be enough to send you over the edge.

✦ Instead of letting the fingers do the walking, use your hips to thrust your pelvis up and down against your digits.

✦ Give the pubic mound a few gentle slaps to wake up the blood and get it flowing.

✦ Including the vagina in the action will make your entire nether regions a supercharged joy center. Lie back and open things wide by holding your lips open with one hand.

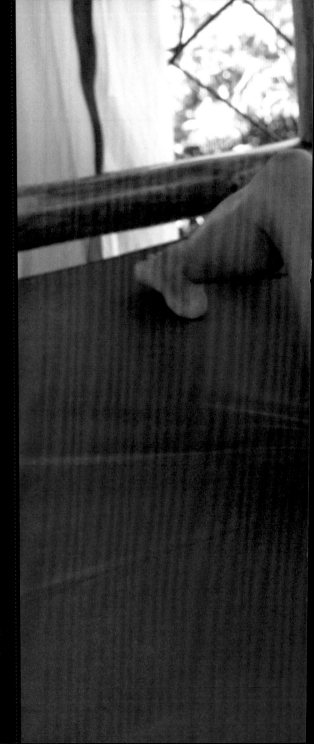

Warm up the entire area using your favorite masturbation Morse code and then get down to biz by slipping an index finger between the labia majora (outer lips) so that it presses against the length of the clitoris. Gentle but firm wrist movements will make the inserted finger rub the clitoris up and down, side to side, and in a circular motion. You can speed things up by doubling the pressure as you begin to get hot under your hood. Crossing your legs and squeezing your thigh muscles together will help you blow your gasket in record time.

◈ To stir up new sensations, rest the palm of your hand on your pubic mound and press down while moving your hand side to side, up and down, and around. A few fingers slipped between the lips to lightly pinch the clitoris will have you ready and raring to go.

◈ Slip a well-greased finger into your anus and press lightly.

◈ Give long slow tickles to ultrasensitive thin-skinned areas like the inner thighs, neck, earlobes, wrists, temples, or lower belly.

Love Nub

Finally, the central moan zone. There are thousands of variations on this theme, so play with different rhythms and motions. Fingers are ideal tools for learning what type of pressure, speed, and stroke work the best.

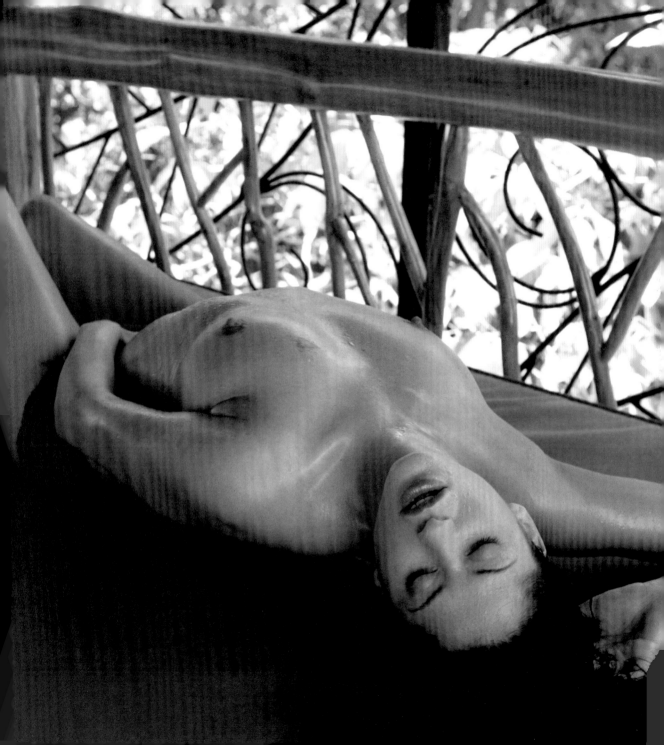

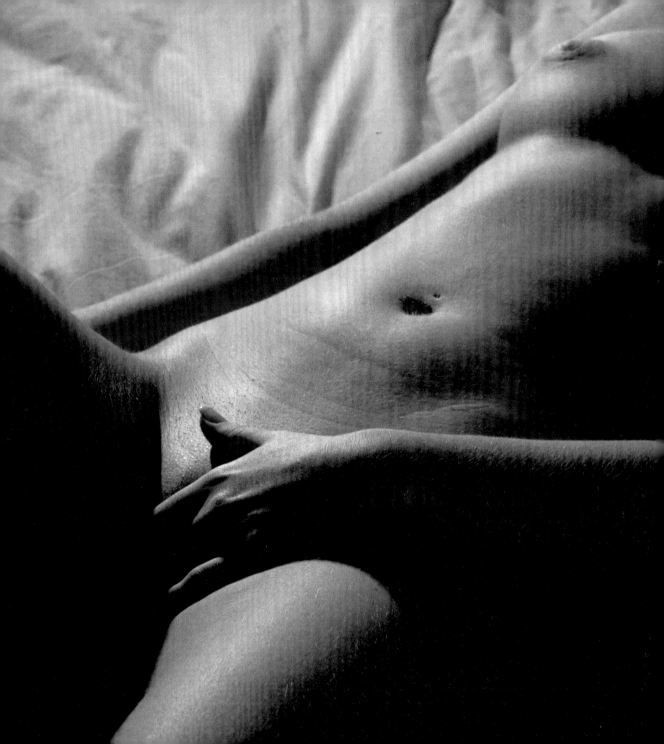

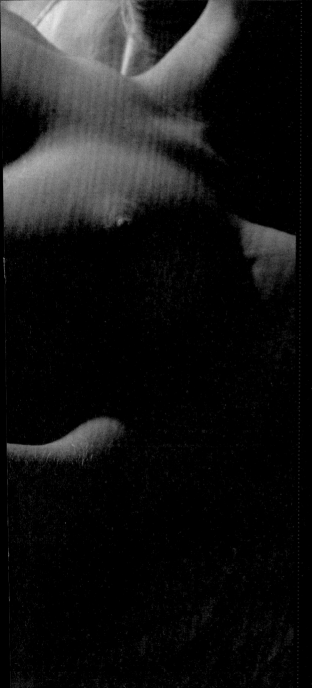

Try a sneak attack Strum away on the whole area and then dive in for the most ticklish bit just before climax. Go slow, using light-as-possible touches to tease and delight—taking note of each move to begin to understand what pleases.

Tried and true Throw in some known feel-good moves such as tracing up and down, in a figure eight, or back and forth; lightly tapping using just one finger; or going in circles on one side or both (switching sides if too much pressure causes numbness in one area), increasing the tempo as arousal builds.

The whole you-bang You can try zigzagging with one or more fingers around the entire zone or, holding fingers in a downward *V*, rub the area straight up and down. Use two fingers of one hand to open the "curtains" and give the index finger of the other hand quick and easy access to the star attraction.

Pinch Hitters

Some women use hairbrush handles, blankets, towels, vegetables, the blunt end of an electric toothbrush, cell phones set on vibrate, the washing machine during spin cycle, hot dogs—basically, anything goes. You should just make sure whatever you use is clean, easy to remove, and not plunged in deep. No one wants to wind up in the ER with a turkey leg stuck in her vagina. Your safest bet is to stick with tools designed for the work.

Dildos These penis-shaped gadgets, some of them exact replicas of the real deal, come in quite handy for women who want to blast their own G-spot or are talented multitaskers able to penetrate themselves while stimulating their clitorises. Some women like to use an object close in shape and size to their partner's tool so they can discover which angles and thrusting styles will hit their hot spots during a doubles match.

Vibrators These trusty joysticks do everything a dildo can, with amps. Some women say it's the only way to go if you have long fingernails. Best for playing with on your own are the short, curved ones that are shaped for stimulating the G-spot and the long, thin ones perfect for zeroing in on areas deep in the vagina. Although vibrators are not as versatile as fingers, the advantage is that they do all the work—all you have to do is lie back and think *bliss*. This makes them ideal for women who just want to have a quick Oh!—as well as those who are gluttons for prolonged pleasure.

Panties on You may want to keep your panties on when you start buzzing, as the sensation can be intense. You can tease yourself by alternating speeds as your desire builds. Try pressing the head against or near the clitoris. Depending on the shape, you can lie down on top of it, lie on your side and prop it up against your love button, or hold it between your legs while lying on your back—leaving your hands free for other things.

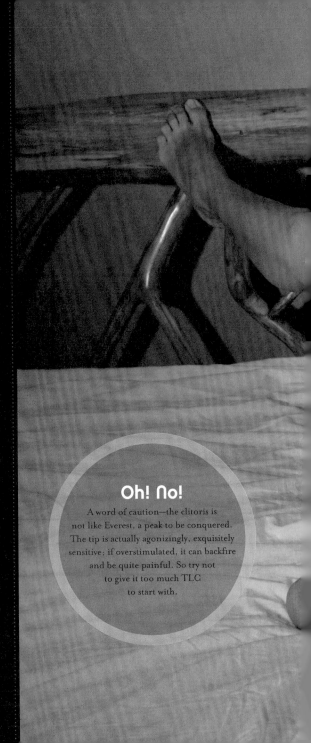

Oh! No!

A word of caution—the clitoris is not like Everest, a peak to be conquered. The tip is actually agonizingly, exquisitely sensitive; if overstimulated, it can backfire and be quite painful. So try not to give it too much TLC to start with.

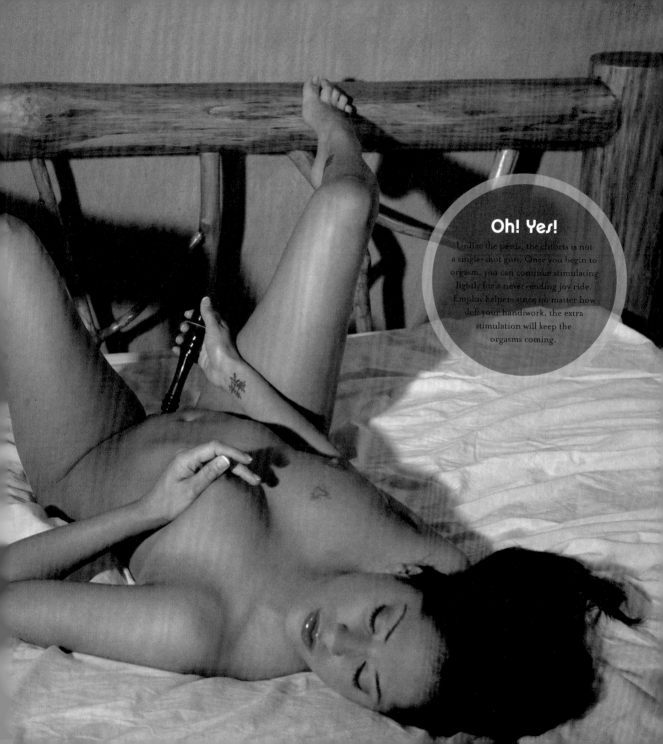

Oh! Yes!

Unlike the penis, the clitoris is not a single-shot gun. Once you begin to orgasm, you can continue stimulating lightly for a never-ending joy ride. Employ helpers since no matter how deft your handiwork, the extra stimulation will keep the orgasms coming.

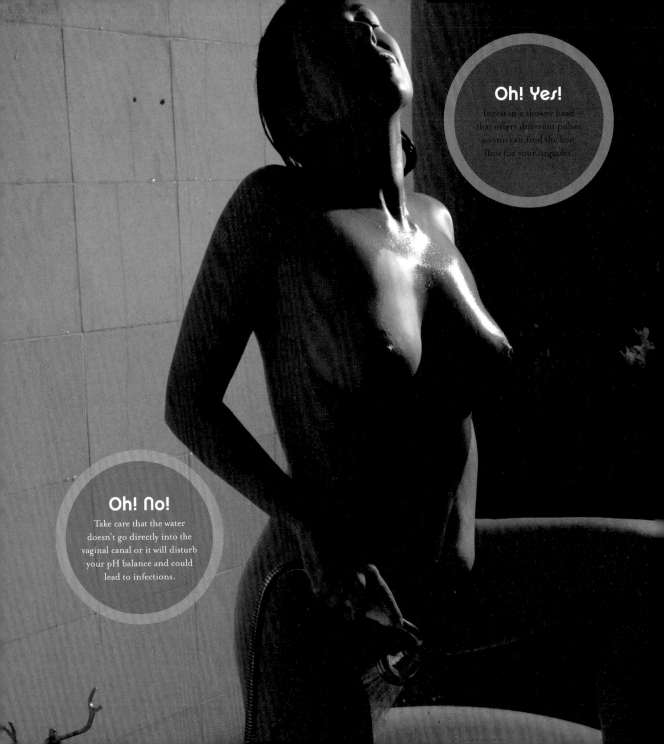

Oh! Yes!

Invest in a shower head that offers different pulses so you can find the best flow for your orgasms.

Oh! No!

Take care that the water doesn't go directly into the vaginal canal or it will disturb your pH balance and could lead to infections.

Water Play

The extra heat from water can be great, but make sure the water isn't too hot for the sensitive skin of the vagina. You can always adjust the temperature once you start heating things up. One supersex secret is to alternate between hot and cold water.

Shower head   A detachable model is the most versatile, but with a little careful positioning, you should be able to aim any shower head to let the water spray over your breasts, belly, and between your legs. The closer you can get it to your body, the more direct and intense the feeling; moving it farther away will cover a larger area and bring on a tubful of different sensations.

Bathtub   The most common position is lying back and letting the water from the faucet wash over the vagina. This isn't always the easiest of positions to stay in, especially if the water is high, so fill the tub only about halfway. You can then lie on your back and bring your bottom up so it's against the end of the tub with the faucet. This will give you room to maneuver your vagina almost directly below the water stream. You might have to tilt your pelvis up to bring your vagina closer.

Jacuzzi/hot tub   Because the sensations are below the surface, you can start with a full immersion and ease into the jets pulsating against your body. When you're ready, turn toward the stream and position your clitoris so it's directly in the path of the flowing water. (But not too close—the pressure is usually strong.)

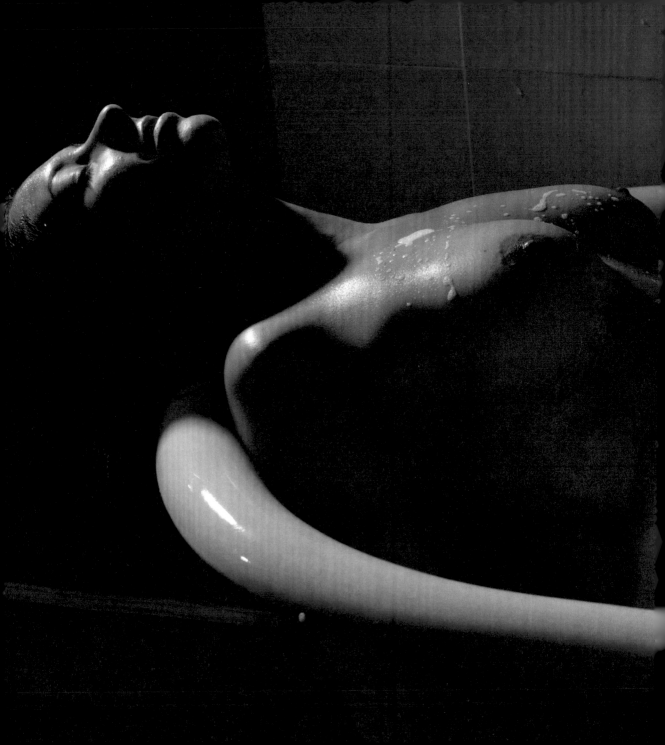

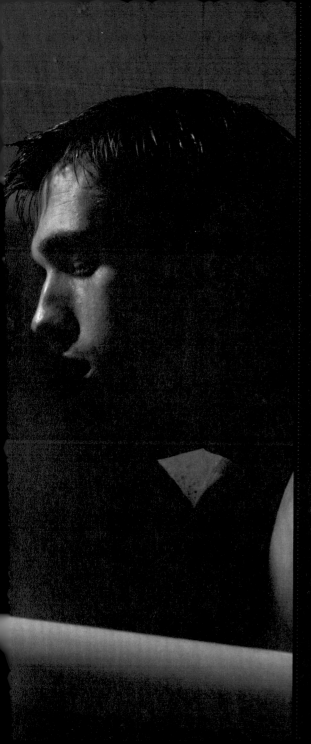

Invite Him to the Party

Mutual masturbation is just another way to say "quickie." Once you're breathing heavy, you can skip straight to sex or finish yourselves off. To take the awkwardness out of the affair, start by kissing each other and then shift the action to solo moves.

This may feel a bit strange. After all, most people are used to trying not to get caught in the act of self-love. But sharing favorite solo moves can let a partner know what makes your body tick—and tock—and tingle. All it takes to turn solo sex into teamwork is four easy steps. But if that still seems too much, don't sweat it. Just playing with herself gives a woman frisky confidence. Four easy steps are all it takes to turn solo sex into teamwork.

1. Get started before he comes—to the door. About an hour before you get together with your partner, play a little. Masturbating until you are almost there will keep you squirming.

2. Talk dirty. If you're too shy to call it out while he's there, you can text him while pleasuring yourself and give him a play-by-play of what you're doing. Think of it as a two-for-the-price-of-one move—it's both a turn-on and an education. Once you and he are actually messing around, put his hand exactly where you want it and murmur how good it feels.

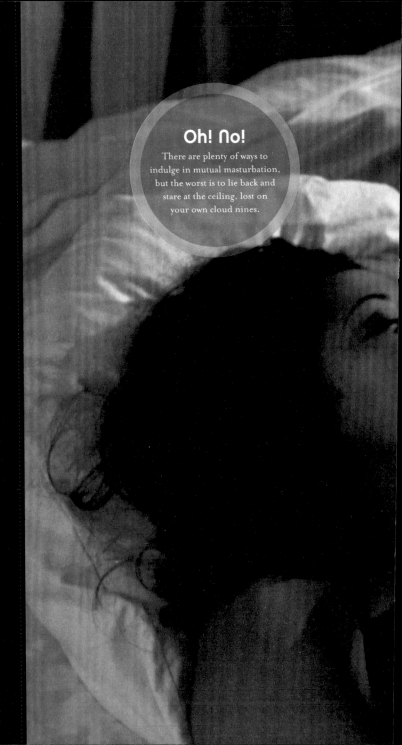

3. Follow the leader. You can skip the cheap talk and simply keep your hand on top of his and move it how you want. A bolder move is to do the same with his tool. Once he catches on, you can let go of him so he can take the steering wheel (encouraged by your groans of appreciation) before you make a different randy request. Or you can reverse the above and let him rest his hand on yours as you take care of your own business.

4. Let him watch. You're guaranteed to have his full attention when you get handy with yourself. He may forget to take notes, but he will get a good sense of what makes you go tra-la-la.

Oh! No!

There are plenty of ways to indulge in mutual masturbation, but the worst is to lie back and stare at the ceiling, lost on your own cloud nines.

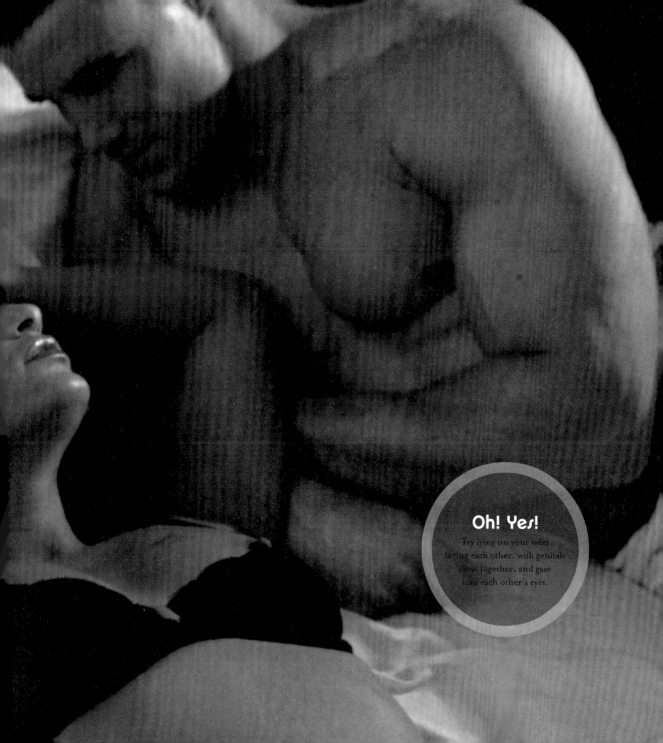

Oh! Yes!

Try lying on your sides
facing each other, with genitals
close together, and gaze
into each other's eyes.

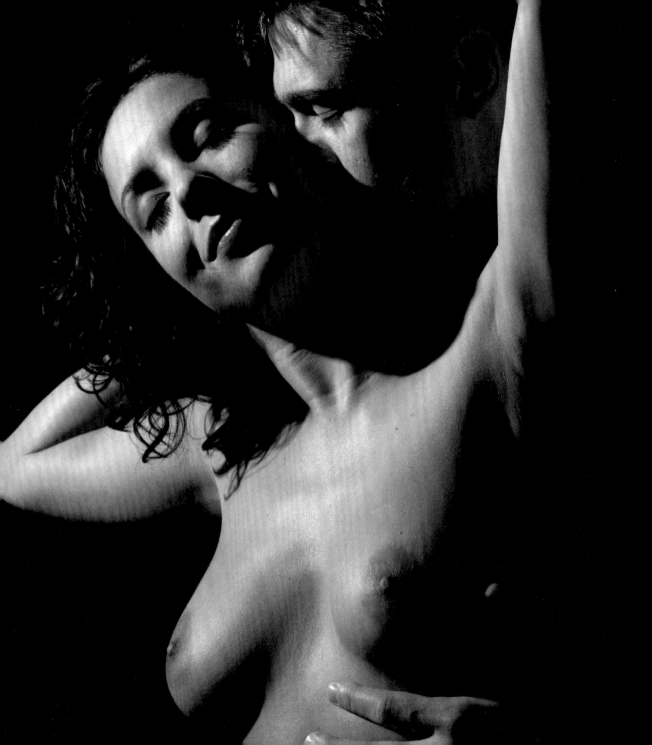

3: GETTING HANDY

Foreplay is so much more than a warm-up to nookie. It's the stuff that turns good sex into phenomenal, bed-shaking, body-quaking sex. The key is to strive for quality—not quantity.

One of the biggest complaints from women on the foreplay front is that their partners zero right in on their goods and spend little or no time exploring other parts of their bodies. This is a shame, because there are plenty of other delectable bits he can touch, tickle, and lick that will rock your world (and his). By taking the time to savor every tantalizing touch, even a caress on the arm might make you whimper.

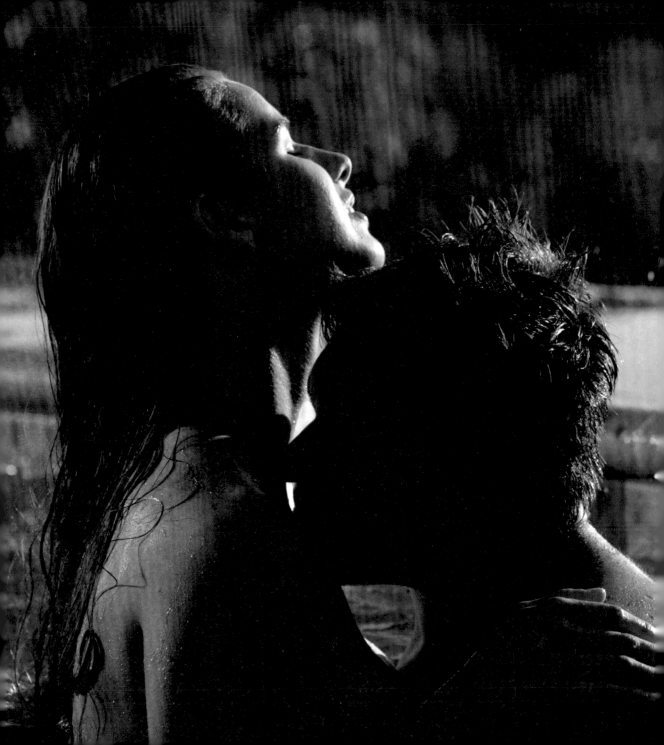

Discover Your Hot Spots...

Almost foreplay   Instead of actually giving you the direct touches you lust for, he should build your anticipation by getting close to your yearn-and-burn places with his hands or mouth and then—whoops!—passing right by. By the time he actually touches you, you'll be primed to detonate.

Shake it up   Even when you're returning to favorite spots, do things differently. If your usual routine is working from the top down, darting around your bliss bits will keep you both delightfully on the erotic edge. Or simply have him slip a blindfold on you to keep you guessing where he'll strike next.

Use his power tool   His penis doesn't come with just two settings, stiff and thrust. You can rub it along the backs of your legs, slide it into your cleavage or along the crease in your bottom, press it into your nipples, or even push it up against the often-overlooked underarm hot spot.

No hands   Touch tends to take over with foreplay, but for the kind of action that causes a nuclear reaction, you need to get all of your senses in on the game—using the eyes, ears, nose, and tongue.

Mouth, breasts, nipples, bottom, vagina—these are most women's usual go-to places for getting steamy. But your body is one big erogenous zone begging to be loved. Everyone has one secret, undiscovered spot that sends them through the roof. Some surprising spots that will make you unhinged:

- Stroking the backs of knees
- Licking the length of the neck and chin
- Lightly scratching where arms and legs join the body
- Massaging between the toes
- Pushing with the entire palm against the sacrum (where your lower back meets your bottom)
- Using the side of the hand to lightly chop the shoulder blades
- Nuzzling the earlobes
- Pressing against the temples
- Rubbing the area above the eyebrows with thumbs
- Grazing the inside of the earlobe
- Sucking on the fingers
- Licking and then blowing on the forearms

Getting Lippy

Mouth-to-mouth tricks that will get you puckering up:

❖ Start soft and then gradually build up to hard, rough, raw kisses.

❖ Don't just kiss—tantalize and tease by tracing the outside of your lips with your tongues, gently tugging at your bottom lips with your teeth, and lightly biting and sucking hard on each other's tongues

❖ Play with the temperature and sip something hot or suck something icy cold right before you lock lips.

❖ Don't limit making out to the lips—put your whole body in on the act by pressing your chests against each other, grabbing at bottoms, and grinding pelvises.

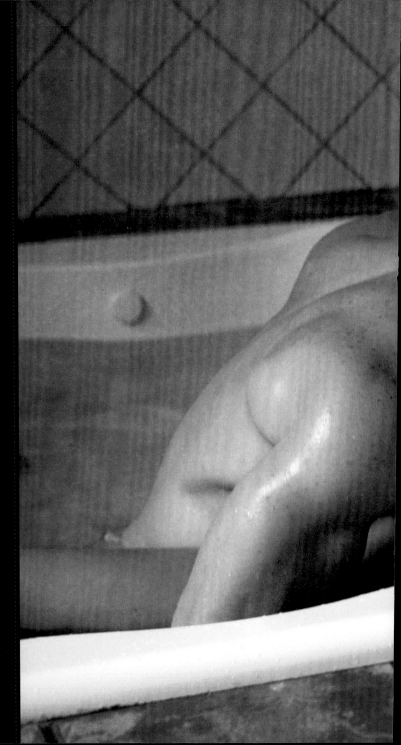

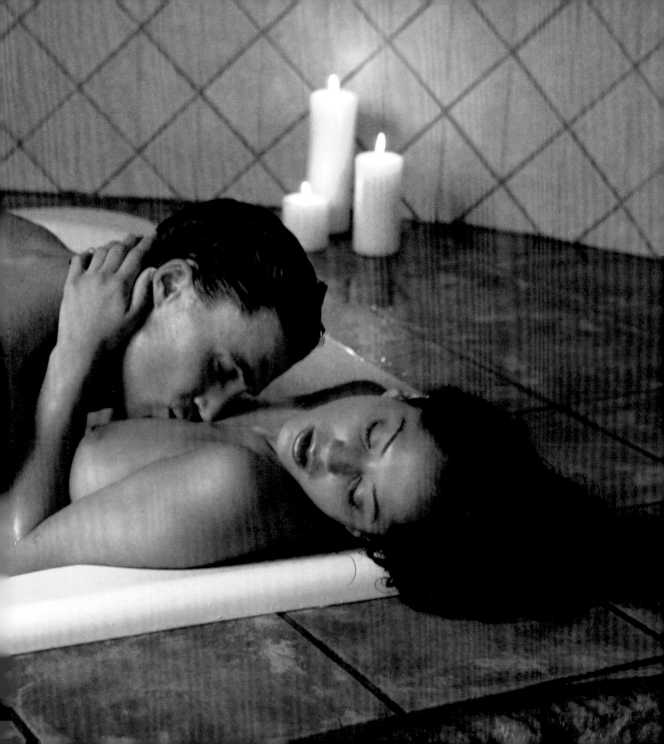

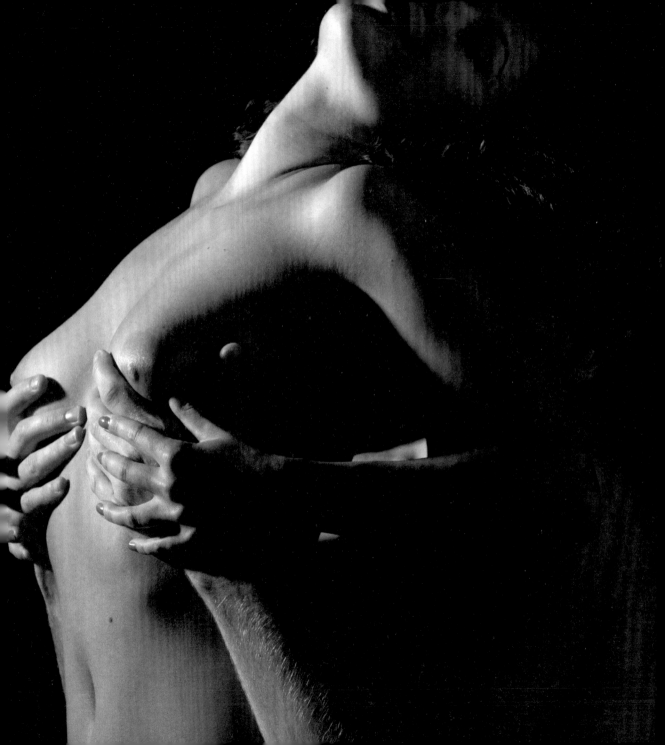

Conquer Your Alps

Instead of limiting himself to the nipples, he can cup the area with his entire hand and gently squeeze. The nerve-rich erogenous tissue on the top, sides, and underside of the breast can actually be more sensitive than an unaroused areola and nipple and will thrill to the lightest touch. Or he can use just one finger to lightly flick your nubs. The nipple (which, like the clitoris, feeds into orgasm-inducing neurons in the brain) loves friction, and the longer it's teased, the more intense direct stimulation will be. But be careful: The nipple can be hypersensitive, so pressure should be applied lightly.

His best overall boob move is to warm things up first by gently massaging your breast with his thumb and index finger and then placing his hand over your areola and rolling it with his palm. Finally, he very gently pulls and teases your nipple.

He can customize his tour of your top half by taking advantage of your size. The smaller the breasts, the more sensitive they feel. Minis also make it easier for him to cup one in his entire hand and gently squash and squeeze. Supersized breasts, on the other hand, have a multitude of hot zones. The best way for him to reach them is for you to lie flat on your back. This will push your breasts up and out, opening them up to his touch.

To up the erotic ante, he can try these nip tips.

❖ Adjust the temperature by mixing in some icy and heated ingredients. Have him put a dollop of ice cream on your nipples, take a slug of whiskey, and then lick it off. The warming liquid in his mouth will make you sweat.

❖ He lightly brushes the very tops of your nipples with just the tips of his index fingers, first trying both together and then one at a time.

❖ He does the same thing, but uses his tongue this time.

❖ He gently rolls your nipples between his thumb and index finger.

❖ Instead of just squeezing, he also pinches and pulls those babies.

❖ He grips each nipple firmly between two fingers and rapidly flicks the tips with his tongue.

❖ He takes the whole nub in his mouth and licks it with the flat of his tongue.

Pass Your Barrier

When it comes to below-the-belt action, he can curl his fingers to brush back and forth between your vagina and clitoris or alternate rotating them over the area clockwise, then counterclockwise. Two fingers are better than one, and four or five are even better.

These tip-you-over techniques to drive your love nub crazy will have a bed-rocking, toe-clenching payoff. Get him to try one for a few minutes, then switch to another. The unpredictability of his teasing will leave you gasping for air. Fingers also make great stand-ins for dildos and, in some ways, are even better than his real organ because they can bend in ways his trusty tool can't for loads of lusty up-the-canal exploration once he's got you going.

A word of warning for him before you start: Many men do wrong by the clitoris because they go straight for the head-on stimulation. This sort of direct touch can actually be painful. It's much better to rub the clitoral hood (where the tops of the labia meet) or to rub along the side of the clitoris.

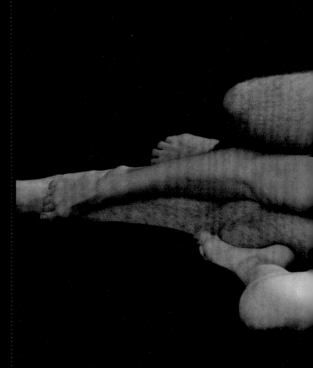

◈ Pressing his thumb against the base of your clitoris, where it meets the pubic bone, will make it even more sensitive, if you can bear it.

◈ The top edge of the clitoris is slightly less sensitive and responds to broader moves

Oh! No!

Because a penis responds very differently than a clitoris to direct stimulation, men tend to follow their own fast pace when giving you a hand job. But women prefer a slow buildup during manual stimulation.

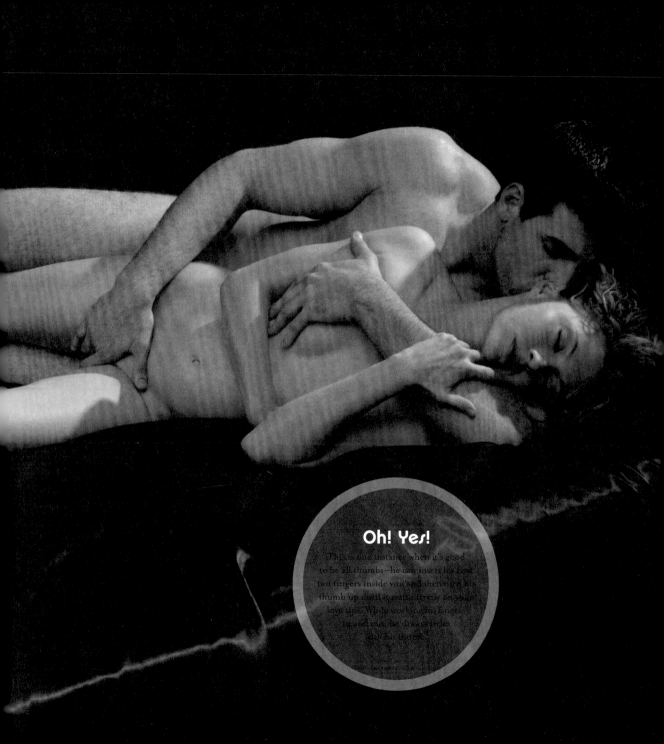

Oh! Yes!

This is one instance when it's good to be all thumbs—he can insert his first two fingers inside you and then nudge his thumb up until it rests directly on your love tips. While working his fingers in and out, he draws circles with his thumb.

such as pressing against it with the heel of the hand and making firm circular movements, always pushing gently downward.

❖ Using his index finger, he traces circles around the base of the clitoris without touching it. At last, he touches it lightly by first drumming with feather-light touches and gradually rapping more sharply and rapidly.

❖ He brushes his finger from side to side along the top of your clitoris.

❖ He uses the thumb of one hand to hold back the hood of the clitoris, gently rubbing the base at the same time. If he's ambidextrous, he can stroke the sides and tip with his other fingers.

❖ He gently rolls the shaft between his thumb and middle finger. Still grasping the shaft, he strokes up and down with his index finger in long, gliding strokes.

❖ He encircles the whole clitoris with the thumb, index finger, and middle finger of one hand and ever so gently tugs.

❖ Now he can try all the above using his tongue or alternating between his tongue and fingers.

❖ The clitoris is sensitive enough to respond to action that's off-site as well.

He can try massaging your love nub through your outer labia (the lips) or brushing his fingers over it through your underwear.

❖ When you're on an orgasm cliffhanger, he can use two fingers to lightly but firmly press against the tip of your clitoris to push you over.

❖ He can drive you wild by working it from all angles, moving in a figure-eight motion to the right, left, right, and left to bring him back where he started. Once he has the pattern down, he can play around with pressure and speed.

❖ Holding the clitoris between his thumb and index finger, he rolls, rolls, rolls, your boat, gently down the stream. Merrily, merrily, merrily, merrily, your orgasm will be a scream.

❖ When time is tight, he can try a C rubdown by holding your clitoris in place with one hand and rubbing in a circular motion with the other. He can easily vary the speed and pressure to suit your time schedule. (Some women orgasm in under a minute with this method.)

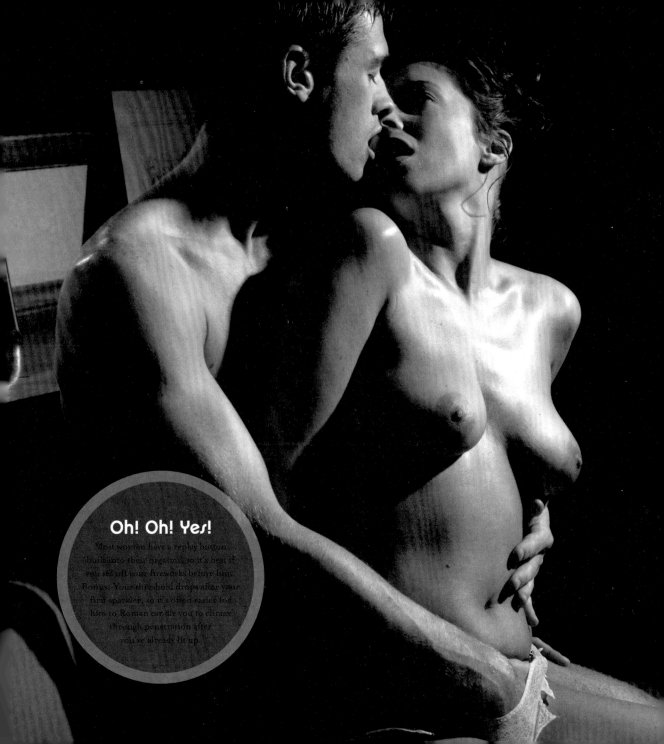

Oh! Oh! Yes!

Most women have a replay button
built into their orgasms, so it's best if
you set off your fireworks before him.
Bonus: Your threshold drops after your
first sparkler, so it's often easier for
him to Roman candle you to climax
through penetration after
you've already lit up.

Shake Your Booty

The bottom usually gets a bum's rush when it comes to foreplay. But it's an easy-to-reach hot zone that will definitely boost your buzz.

- Have him get slaphappy. A light spanking and squeezing of your cheeks can make you shiver with delight.

- He doesn't need to go deep to tickle those nervy bits. A well-lubricated finger circling the rim of the anus will make your bottom twitch. Or he can hold his finger flat and rub it back and forth. If that gets either of you hankering for more, feel free to delve deeper.

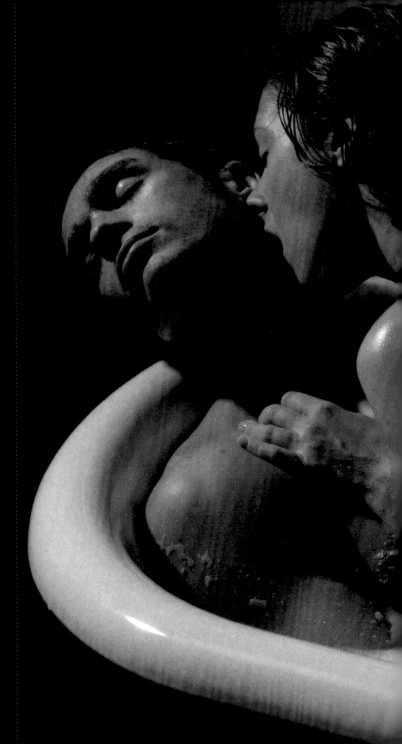

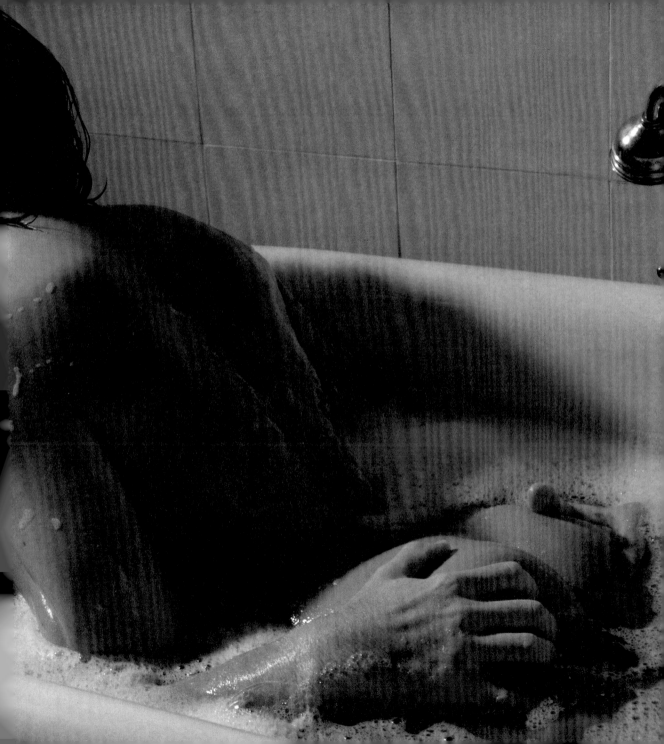

Double Your Fun

Zeroing in on the major erogenous areas is crucial for making you moan for mercy. But to hit your high note even faster, multitask. Any time more than one spot can be stirred up simultaneously, more nerve endings are stimulated. Plus, the separate sensations also create twice the anticipation, which ups allover excitement and pushes you over the edge sooner.

There are plenty of ways he can divvy up the use of his hands or mouth: playing with your breasts while he works south of the border; seeing if his fingers can meet and greet via your front and rear entrances; caressing your neck while stroking your breasts; touching your body all over with fluttery, barely there kisses and strokes.

But you don't need to just lie back and take it. You can also get in on the fun and games, fondling yourself in sync to his moves. It will feel like another lover is in bed with you.

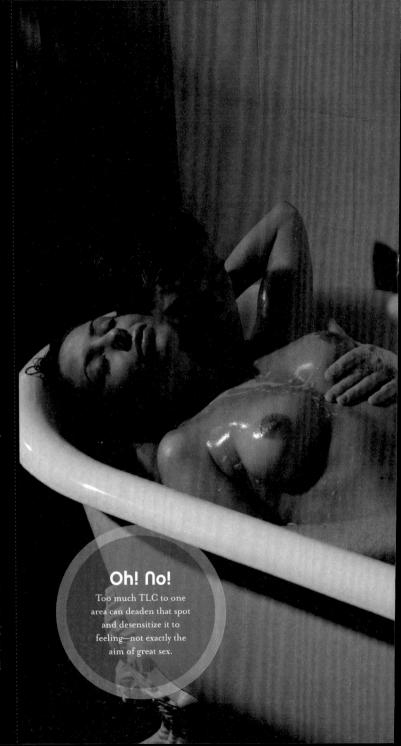

Oh! No!

Too much TLC to one area can deaden that spot and desensitize it to feeling—not exactly the aim of great sex.

Oh! Yes!

Random all-over body teases
keep the action from getting boring.
When you're totally in the moment, your
skin shivers and your muscles tremble
slightly when stroked. When you go
completely still, it's a cue that it's time
to detour those loving attentions to
another part of the body
for a few minutes.

Manhandle Him

Foreplay is not a girly activity.
Given the option, most men would
prefer to play the entire course
than go for a hole in one. All that
pre-sex teasing is just as tantalizing
for him and has the same
anticipation-building booster
effect on his orgasm.

He lusts after all the same
caresses as you—but with less of
a tender touch. Men tend to be
the tougher sex, so go ahead and
push, prod, and pressure him into
passion putty: pinch his nipples
(yes, this is also a red-hot zone for
him), scratch your nails over his
skin, squeeze his bun cheeks, knead
his lower back, dig your fingers
into his waist. Don't worry—he's
strong enough to take it.

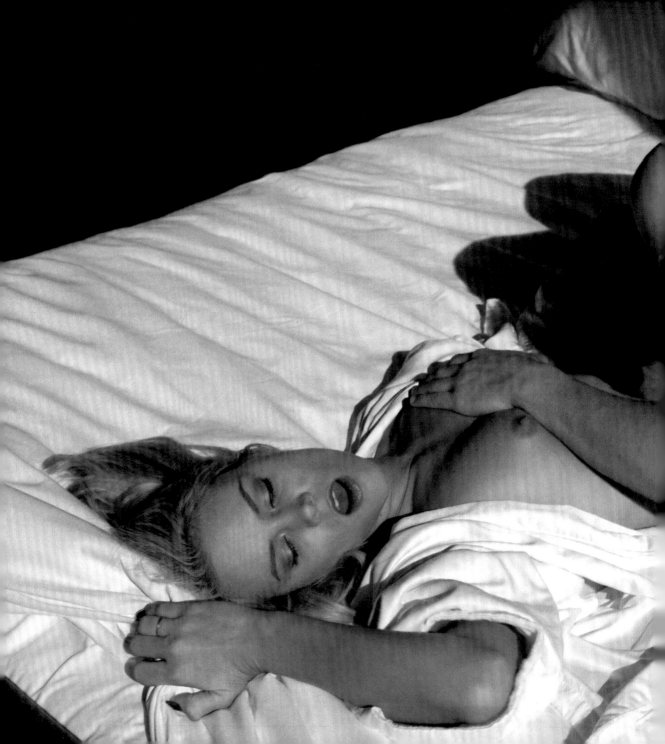

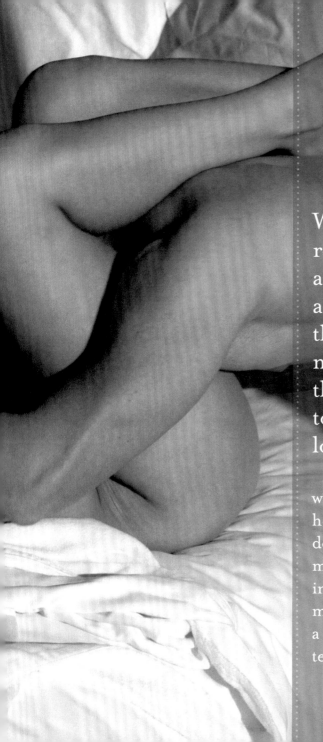

4: MOUTHING OFF

When a woman is on the receiving end of a man's oral attention, she's having really amazing sex—inch for inch, the muscle in his mouth holds more potential for her bliss than the one in his pants. His tongue can deftly get into lusty locales that his penis can't.

Although he can do some pretty wonderful things once it gets there, he shouldn't be in a hurry to head downtown. There's all the rest of your—mmmm, mmmm, good—body to lick into shape. Hands down, the easiest and most delicious way for him to give you a lip-smacking orgasm is to mercilessly tease you with his tongue.

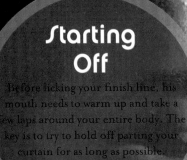

Starting Off

Before licking your finish line, his mouth needs to warm up and take a few laps around your entire body. The key is to try to hold off parting your curtain for as long as possible.

Mouth

Using his mouth to kiss you smack on the lips is an obvious way to get you simmering. The mouth is a major erogenous zone, packed with nerve endings. He can try barely there, light butterfly kisses before heading into a sweep-you-off-your-feet deep smooch.

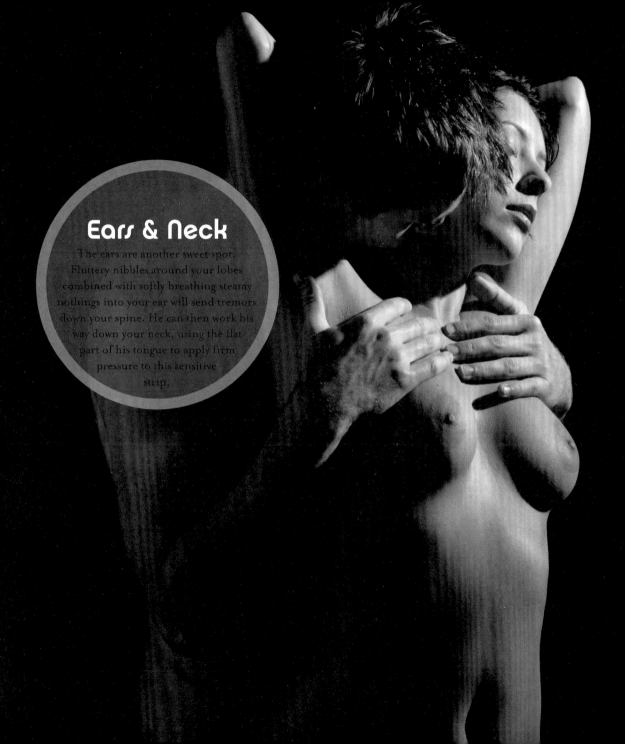

Ears & Neck

The ears are another sweet spot.
Fluttery nibbles around your lobes
combined with softly breathing steamy
nothings into your ear will send tremors
down your spine. He can then work his
way down your neck, using the flat
part of his tongue to apply firm
pressure to this sensitive
strip.

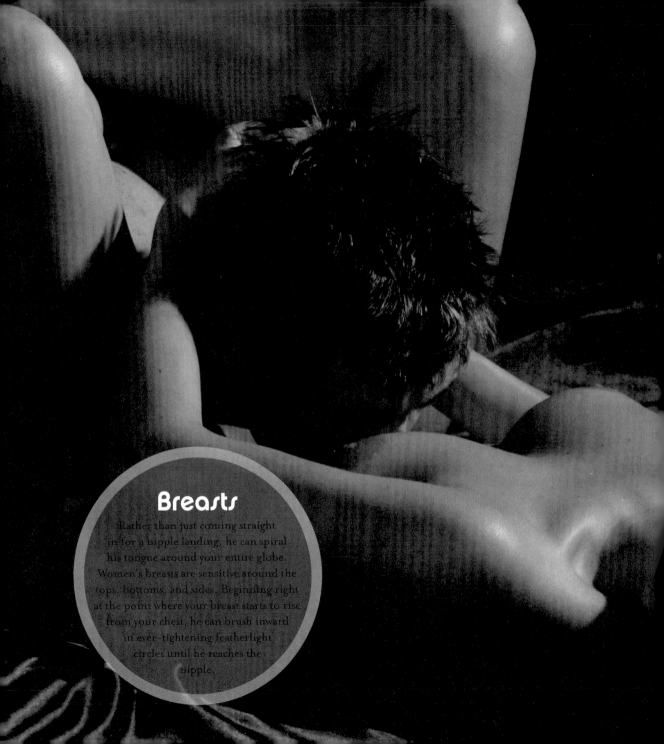

Breasts

Rather than just coming straight in for a nipple landing, he can spiral his tongue around your entire globe. Women's breasts are sensitive around the tops, bottoms, and sides. Beginning right at the point where your breast starts to rise from your chest, he can brush inward in ever-tightening featherlight circles until he reaches the nipple.

Navel

As he heads down, he can tease you by running the tip of his tongue lightly around your belly button. Around three or four finger widths down from the navel is what acupressurists call "The Gate of Origin." Gently pressing down with his tongue on this hot spot will open sexual energy.

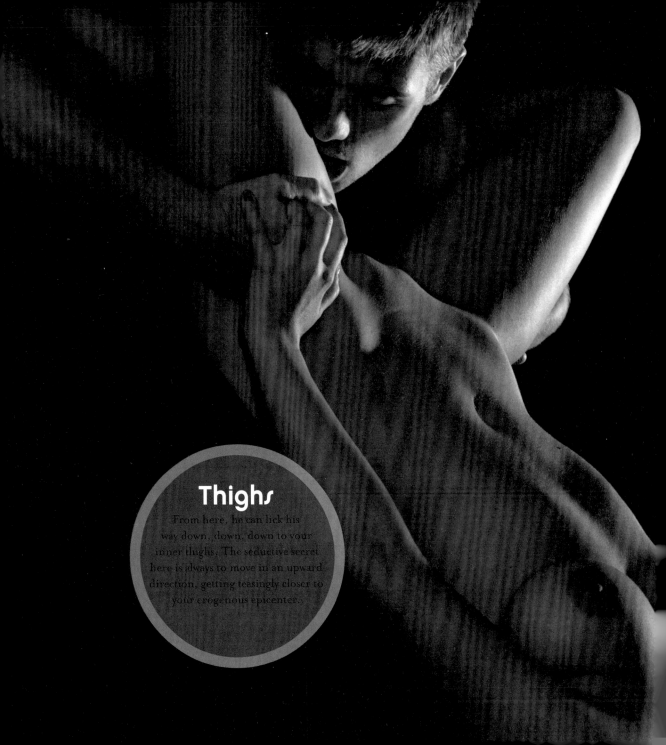

Thighs

From here, he can lick his
way down, down, down to your
inner thighs. The seductive secret
here is always to move in an upward
direction, getting teasingly closer to
your erogenous epicenter.

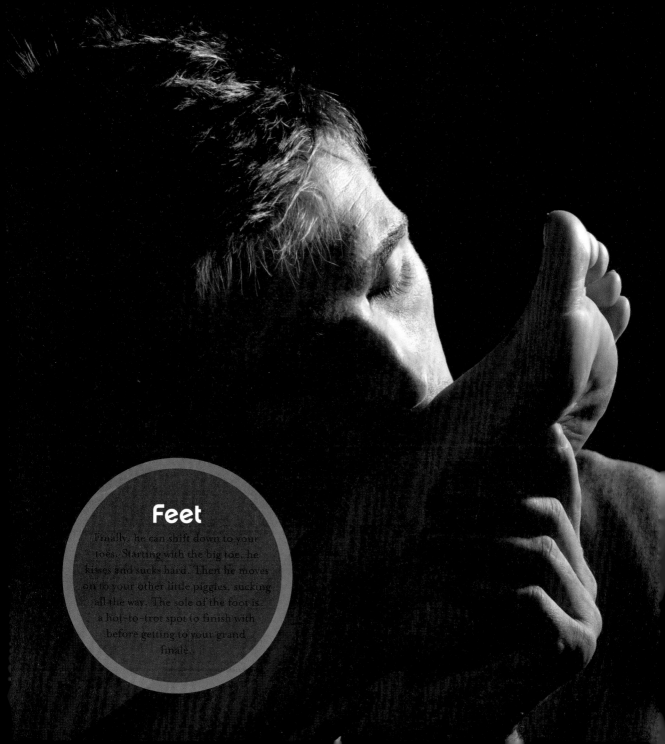

Feet

Finally, he can shift down to your toes. Starting with the big toe, he kisses and sucks hard. Then he moves on to your other little piggies, sucking all the way. The sole of the foot is a hot-to-trot spot to finish with before getting to your grand finale.

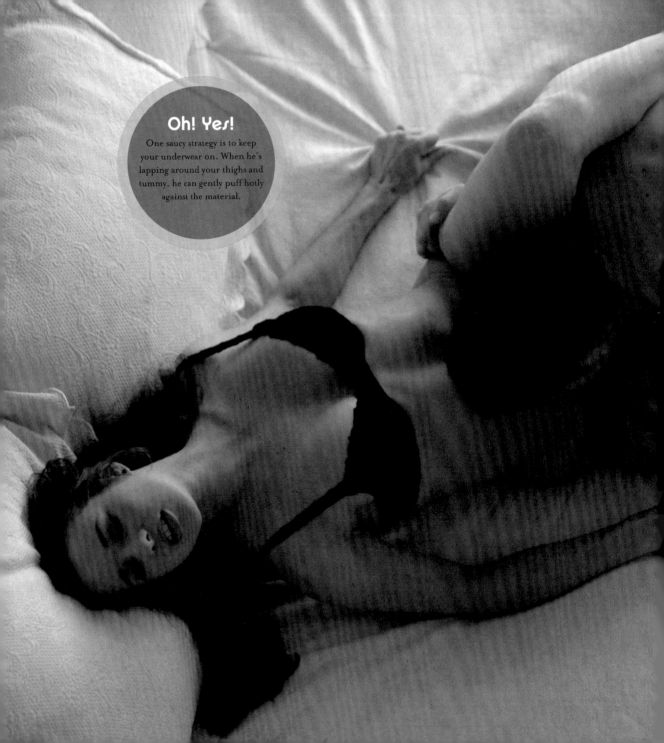

Oh! Yes!

One saucy strategy is to keep your underwear on. When he's lapping around your thighs and tummy, he can gently puff hotly against the material.

Train His Chops

Now he's ready to pay lip service to your private bits. If he isn't sure what you like, he can let you guide him to the right kind of rub by pressing his lips, tongue, or even his chin between your legs and then just lightly holding your hips. You might not take up the challenge right away, but you won't need more than a minute of this slow-mo stimulation to get orgasmically antsy—so take over and push against him in the direction you need him to go.

Alternating among these clitoral tongue twisters is sure to cause an interlude of deluxe delight.

Tongue Tips

Going wide He sticks his tongue out of his mouth so that it's flat, as if he were trying to touch his nose. He can now start lapping you into a frothy lather.

Poke it He points his tongue to press hard and circle it inside his mouth. Now, holding the pose, he does the same between your legs.

Oh! No!

He should never blow air into your vagina. Air forced directly into the vagina, without allowing any to escape, could create an air embolism, which can be fatal.

Floppy   Letting his tongue flop like a sock puppet, he lolls it up and down and back and forth against you.

Licks and Flicks

Lap it up   Leaving his tongue soft and his jaw relaxed, he licks you from your vaginal entrance up to your clit. This is a really good starting caress.

Lock down   He lightly squishes the lips of your vagina together so the inside lip is ever so slightly exposed. He then runs his tongue along one side. Repeat on the other side.

Tongue sex   He pokes his tongue in and out like a mini penis.

The wag   He spreads your lips wide with his fingers and flicks a pointed stiff tongue firmly against your love knob.

The slurpy   Placing his lips over your clitoris, he sucks hard. If he can rub his belly and pat his head at the same time, then he'll be able to work his tongue into the action and press down so that he's alternating between gentle and strong motions.

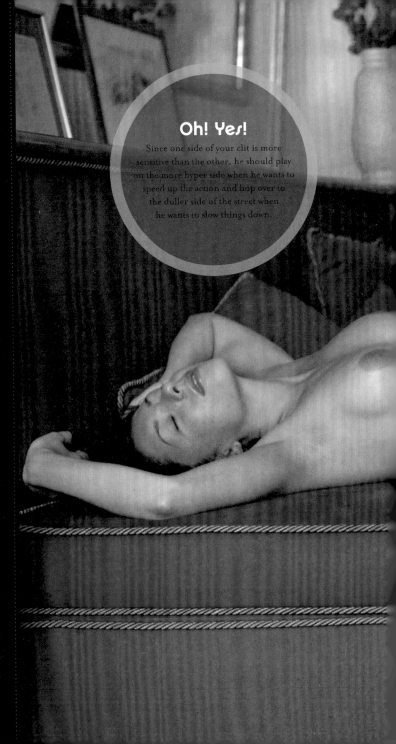

Oh! Yes!

Since one side of your clit is more sensitive than the other, he should play on the more hyper side when he wants to speed up the action and hop over to the duller side of the street when he wants to slow things down.

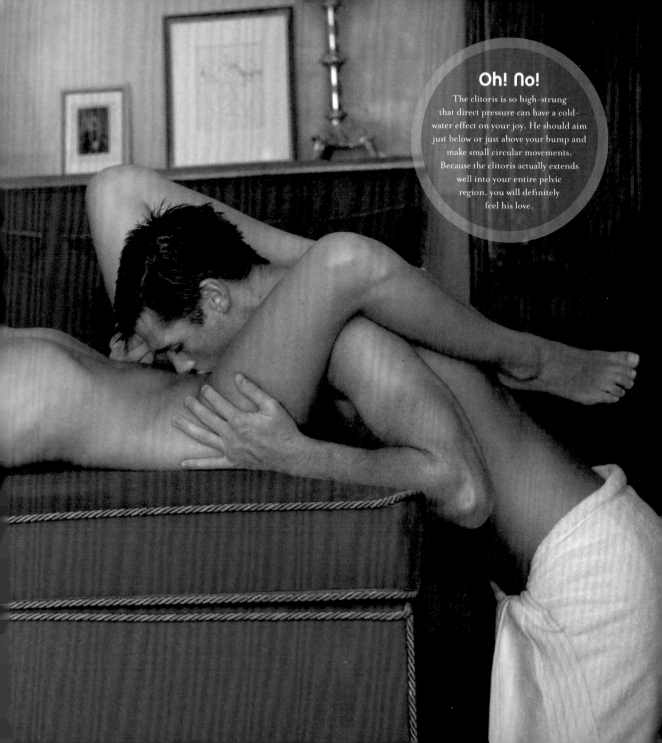

Oh! No!

The clitoris is so high-strung
that direct pressure can have a cold-
water effect on your joy. He should aim
just below or just above your bump and
make small circular movements.
Because the clitoris actually extends
well into your entire pelvic
region, you will definitely
feel his love.

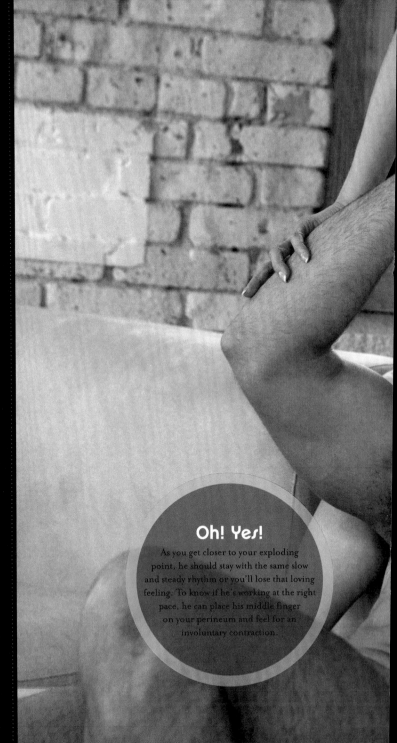

The tube If he can (some people can't), he curls his tongue around your clitoris and slides it back and forth.

O for it He shapes his lips into an *O* and gently sucks on your clitoris.

The switch-hitter He starts with slow, rhythmic, tongue strokes (as if he's licking a popsicle) to get you all worked up. Then, when you start to twitch, he catches your drips with a series of quick, teasing licks.

The love lesson He uses his tongue to spell out the ABCs against your genitals. This keeps his tongue moving in different, unpredictable directions, which keeps you on the edge of your seat.

Rest stop If he needs to catch his breath, he can keep the sensations in a holding pattern by sticking his nose, cheeks, and chin between your legs and waggling them around.

Oh! Yes!

As you get closer to your exploding point, he should stay with the same slow and steady rhythm or you'll lose that loving feeling. To know if he's working at the right pace, he can place his middle finger on your perineum and feel for an involuntary contraction.

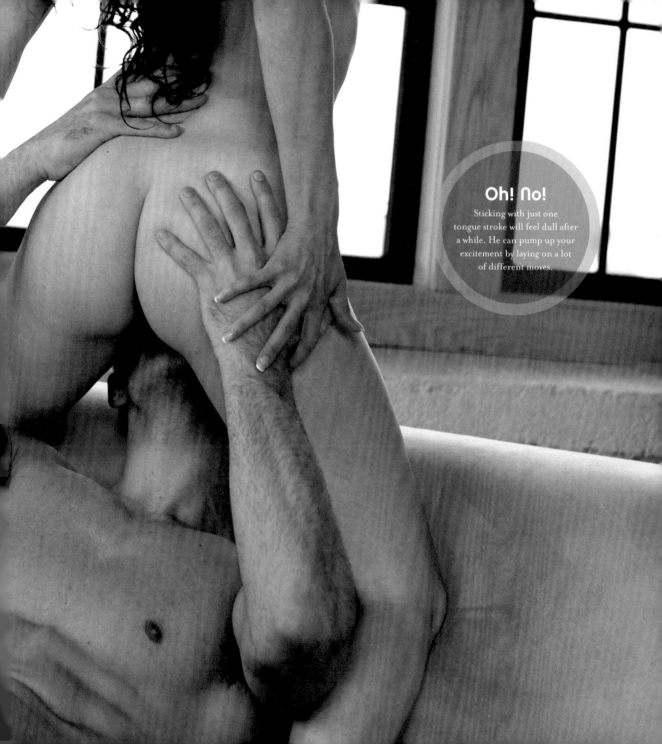

Oh! No!

Sticking with just one
tongue stroke will feel dull after
a while. He can pump up your
excitement by laying on a lot
of different moves.

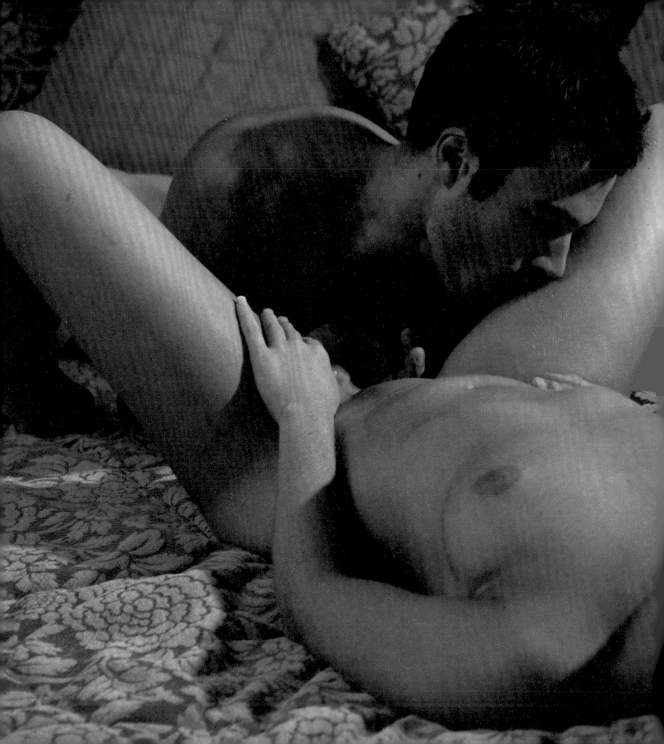

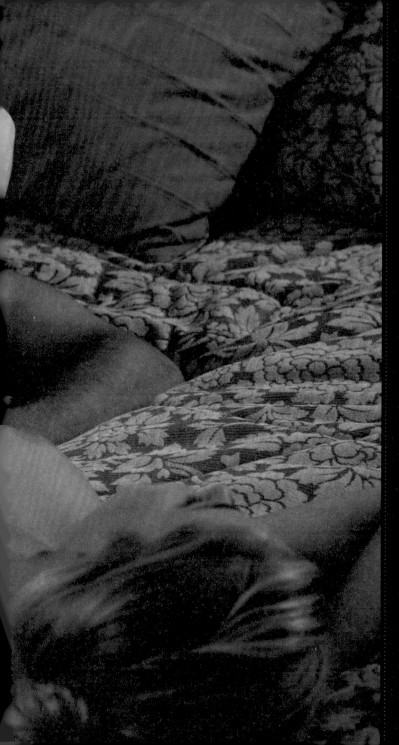

Finger Lickin' Good

Handy moves either of you can use during oral sex to make you twist and shout.

Peace Forming a *V* with the index and middle fingers around your clitoris helps define his lapping ground.

Remove the hood Pulling back the skin of the clitoral head bares the clitoris to his TLC.

Giving the finger Using one or two digits to penetrate you will make you feel like you're taking part in an orgy.

Working the dials Caressing your breasts will instantly triple your happiness quotient.

The Perfect Pose

These access angles give plenty of scope for him to work some mouth magic.

Get stacked   If you're flat on your back, slip a cushion under your hips and another under his chest to ease up your lower back and his neck while making it easier for you to adjust your knees and legs to get the pressure on point.

Get up off it   Keeping his head between your legs can create neck strain. By resting his chin on his fist, he'll be able to give you all the pressure you pine for without unnecessary tension. This also put his fingers right on target for getting in on the action.

Get geometric   Instead of coming at you straight on, have him move in from a right angle. This way, he can stroke his tongue across your clitoris, rather than up and down. It's easier for him, and superintense for you.

Get upside down   Lie crosswise on the bed so that your head is just over the edge—this sends the blood straight to your brain. But make sure the rest of you is stable. When combined with a little nether-region action, this shift in position can cause an orgasmic head rush.

Get lifting   Just before climaxing during oral sex, you can raise your hips slightly and clench your butt muscles to make it more intense.

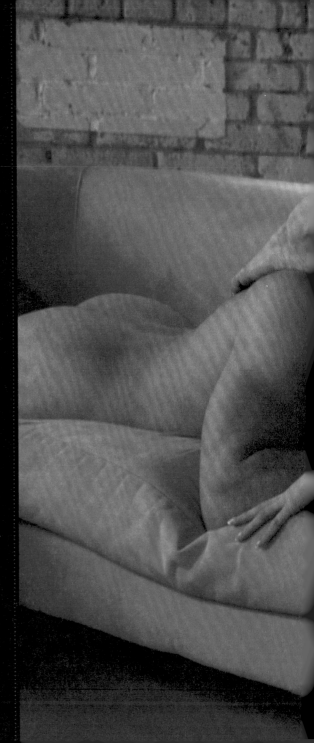

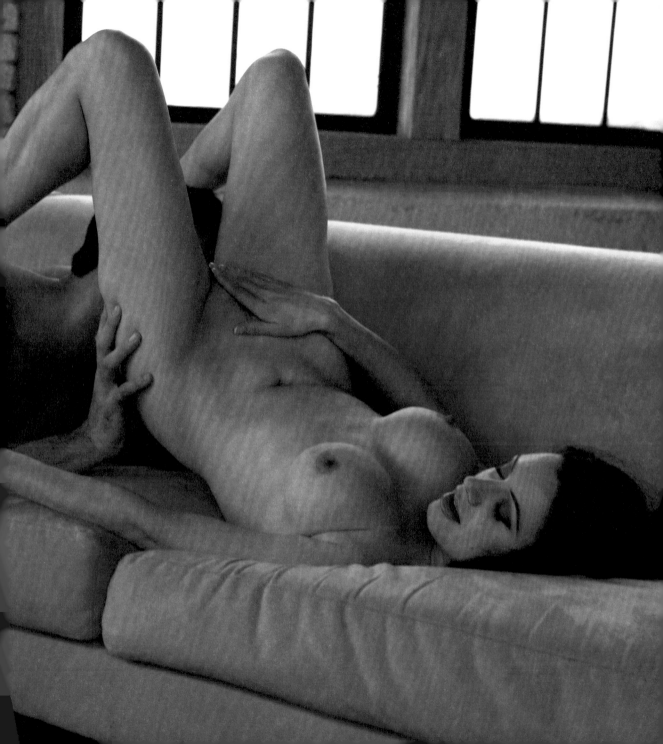

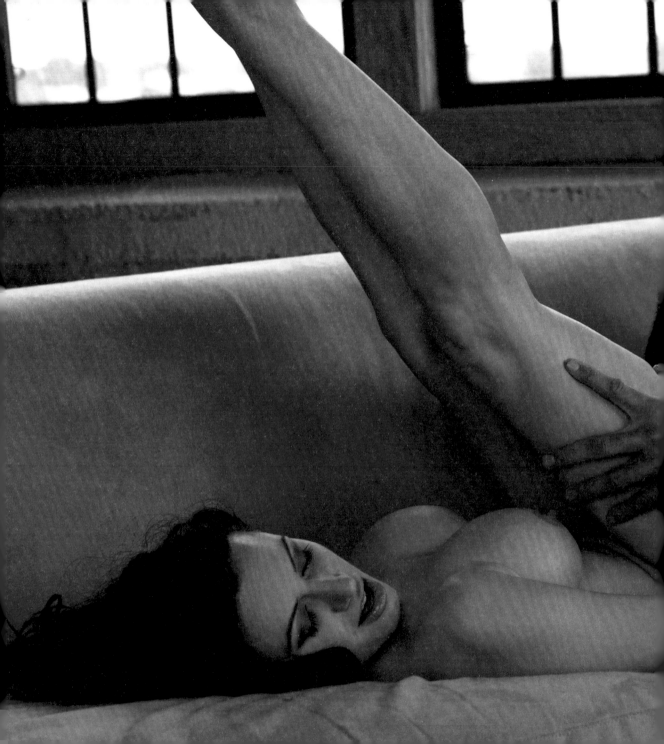

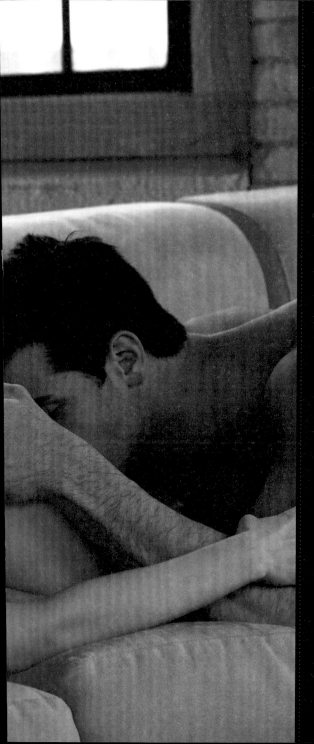

Get out of bed   Moving the action to a chair that has a rocking motion will let you control the rhythm of his licks.

Get him out of there   Keeping your legs closed during oral sex is a tantalizing way to slow him down while teasing yourself silly.

Get a leg up   Pulling one leg up high will completely open you up to whatever sensations he doles out. You can be on your back or your side.

Get over it   If he wants a quick and easy way to figure out your favorite side (clitorally), he can hold one of your legs on his shoulder and the other flat on the bed and give you some loving administrations. You'll instinctively twist your hips in the direction you want him to go.

Get in the back   Although coming at you with his mouth from behind while you're on all fours can restrict his access a bit, it's the perfect pose for hitting bits his tongue might not usually reach in other positions.

Get on it   When he lies back and you straddle his face, you're in complete control of his speed, pressure, and the direction of your delectation. The same goes if you stand with him kneeling in front of you. (Tip: He should hold on to your hips to help you keep your balance at the crucial meltdown moment.)

Get Synched

Couples can harmonize their titillating tune by giving each other a tongue lashing at the same time. It's hard to give and get simultaneously, especially when it comes to pleasure. The secret to a successful 69 is not to be creative. Instead, try to imitate your love organs with your mouths. Have him slide a firm tongue in and out of you like a penis while you hold him between your lips and suck hard. Get into a steady rhythm and keep it up until you both are consumed by mutual ecstasy.

❖ Make beautiful music together by pressing your lips against each other's love regions and gently humming.

❖ Change positions. Side by side is the most popular pose for 69, but it isn't the most effective for mutual satisfaction. The best angle is for your partner to be lying flat on his back with a pillow under his head while you position yourself so that you're bobbing from above. This way, you can control how deep he goes and he can do his moves without any neck strain.

❖ Use delayed starts. Both partners usually don't finish in a dead heat. So it might be a good idea for the favored lover to give the other an oral head start before joining the race.

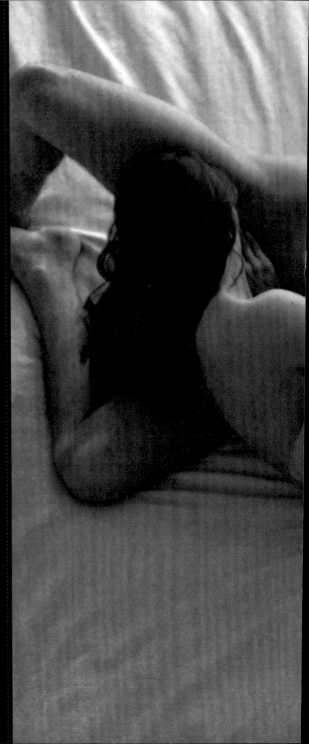

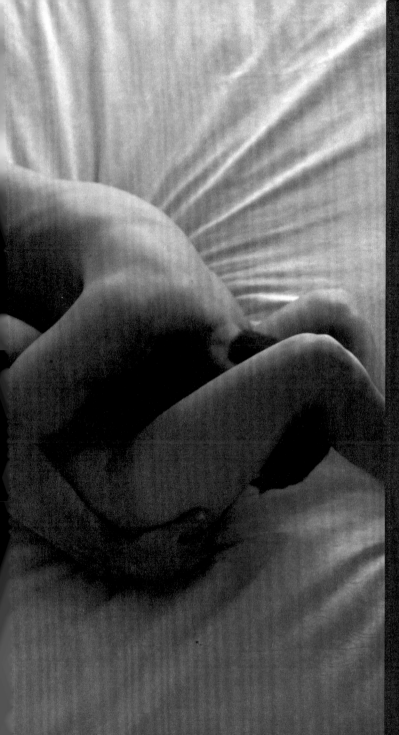

Below-the-Belt Tricks

Blow-by-blow tips for you.

✦ Lick the skin between his balls, then lightly suck each one.

✦ Gently rub a bit of flavored lube onto the head of his penis while licking his shaft with your other hand.

✦ Lift his sac, and flick your tongue on the crease of skin where the scrotum meets his body.

✦ Join your hand and mouth to hold his penis and move them up and down in slow and steady rhythm.

✦ Cradle his penis between your breasts as you lick him.

✦ Lie in missionary position with your head slightly over the edge of the bed to create an ideal deep-throat canal.

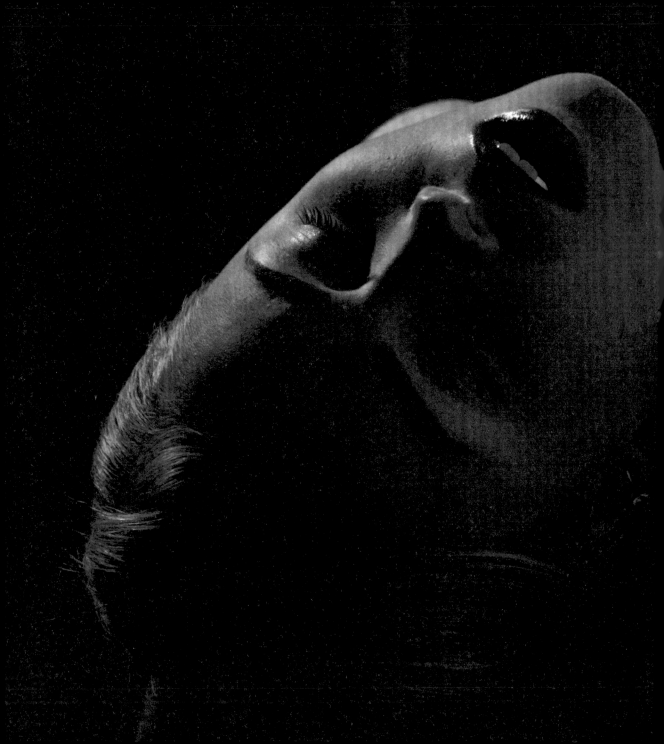

5: ALL THE RIGHT MOVES

The best kind of sex is a combination of passion, pleasure, playfulness, and perspiration. The perfect blend is all in the positioning. In theory, there are thousands of possible sex positions (the *Kama Sutra* lists 529), some of which will put you in a body cast for a month.

Luckily, all it usually takes is a few tweaks to your usual routine to knock your socks off. Put a spin on the four tried-and-true starting positions—missionary, you-on-top, from behind, and side-by-side—with an arm wrapped around him there and a leg flung over your head here and wowza! Get ready to meet your new favorite moves.

Missionary

A few simple tricks will help you take this classic pose from bland to bold. Pillows are your number-one props for taking missionary to the next level. Place one under your bottom or the small of your back to get his pubic bone rubbing up close to your clitoris. Slipping a pillow under your hips will also push him in the direction of your G-spot—the higher you raise your legs, the deeper the penetration against the front wall of your vagina, the more satis-sighing the results.

While you're on the bottom, a sneaking move will get him thrusting deep down into your cul-de-sac before he even knows what hit him. Lift your legs straight up into the air and then back toward your body, and suck in your stomach—the combo of holding in and opening the vaginal canal will give his tool access to your supersensitive spot that you never knew you had.

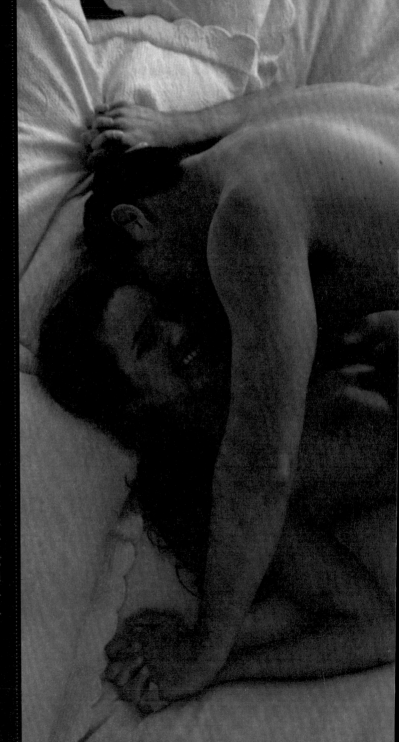

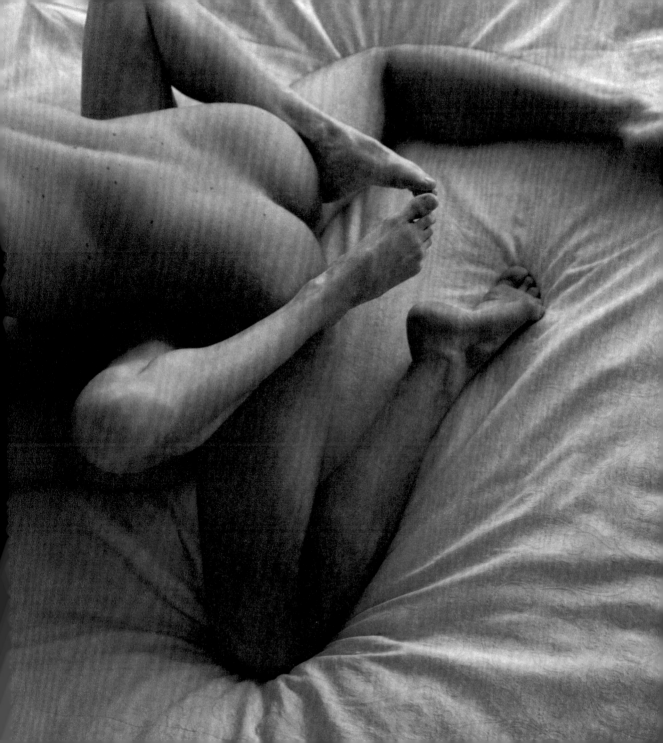

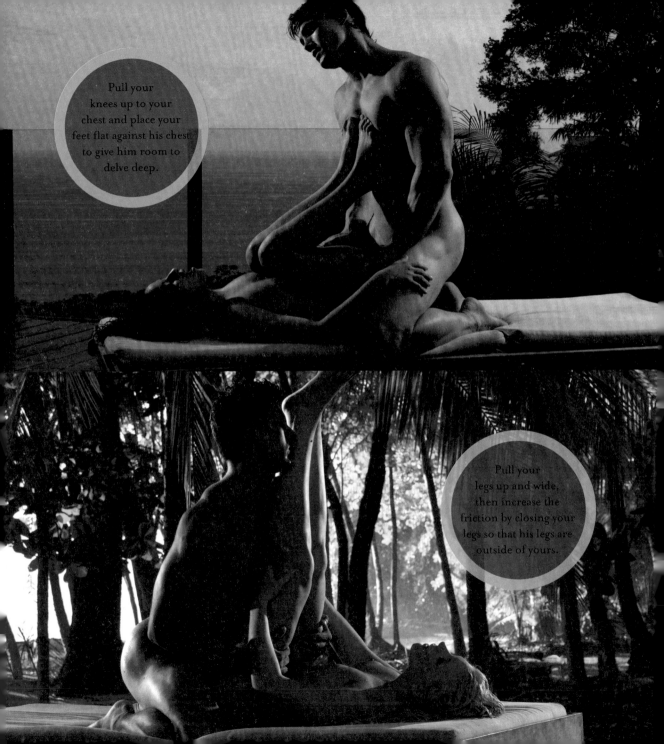

Pull your
knees up to your
chest and place your
feet flat against his chest
to give him room to
delve deep.

Pull your
legs up and wide,
then increase the
friction by closing your
legs so that his legs are
outside of yours.

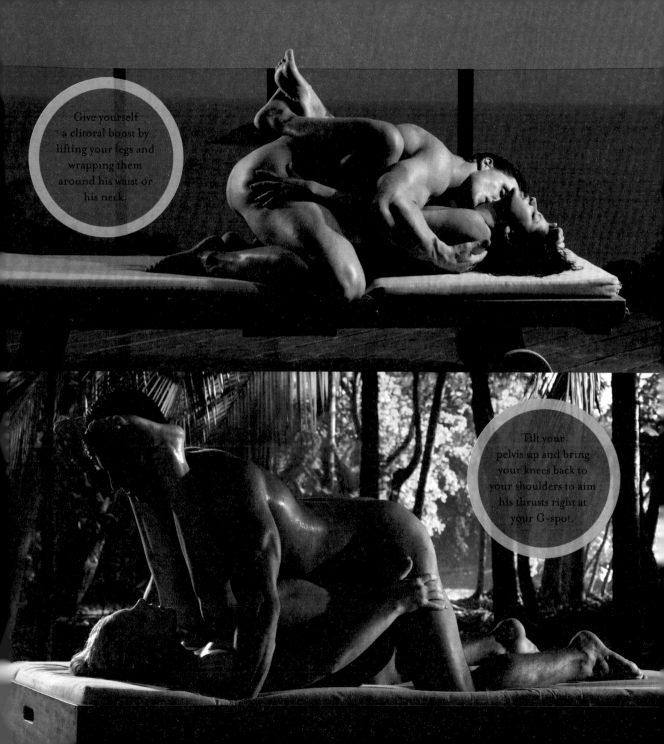

Give yourself a clitoral boost by lifting your legs and wrapping them around his waist or his neck.

Tilt your pelvis up and bring your knees back to your shoulders to aim his thrusts right at your G-spot.

You on Top

Take charge and take care of business (your way!) by climbing into girl-on-top. You can hold a flirtatious look while staying in control of what's exploding down below in all your dynamite spots. This is also the best pose to push tush: He reaches to your backside, grabs onto your globes, and pulls you in tight. Lean back while you straddle him and you're sure to push his penis hard against the front wall of your vagina; then arch your body toward him and you'll double the pleasure as you grind your pleasure point against his pelvis.

The best way to make sure he hits your AFE is to position your body high up on his hips, or tantalize your urethra by staying high on top where you can keep his strokes very shallow, sliding the head of his penis out until it's just nuzzling your vaginal opening and then completely withdrawing it. Keep it up—until he can't. Each new thrust will be like an electric charge.

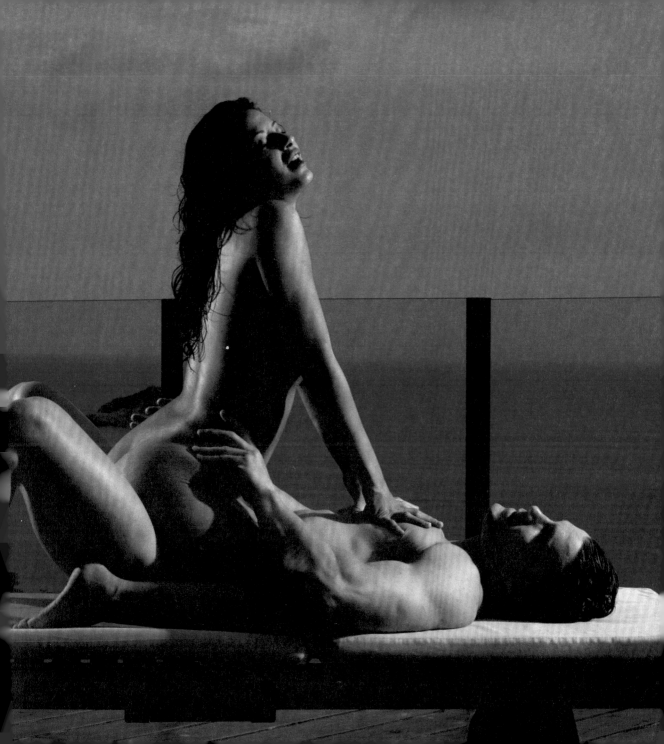

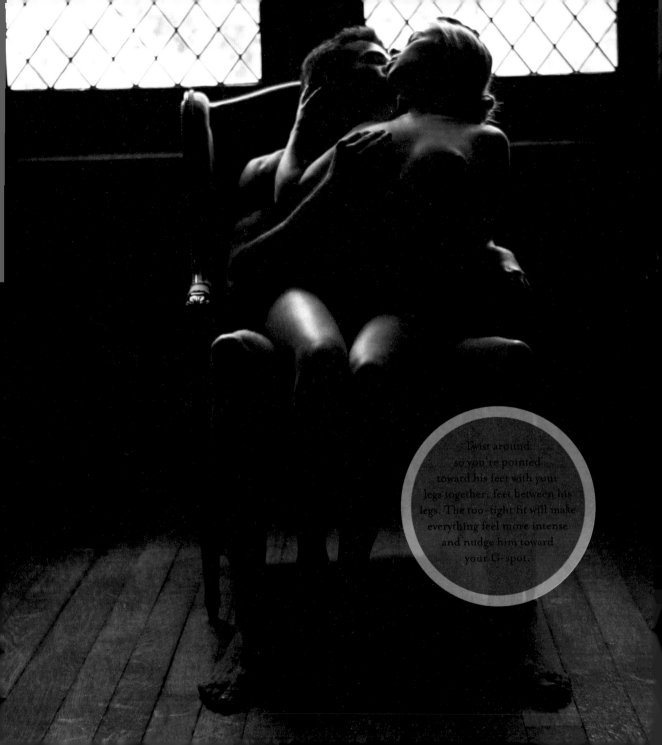

Twist around
so you're pointed
toward his feet with your
legs together, feet between his
legs. The too-tight fit will make
everything feel more intense
and nudge him toward
your G-spot.

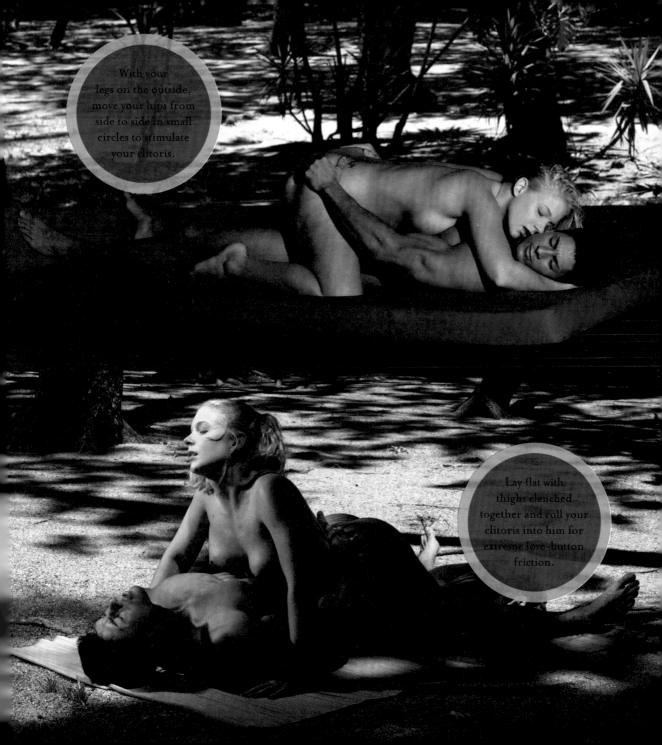

With your legs on the outside, move your hips from side to side in small circles to stimulate your clitoris.

Lay flat with thighs clenched together and roll your clitoris into him for extreme love-button friction.

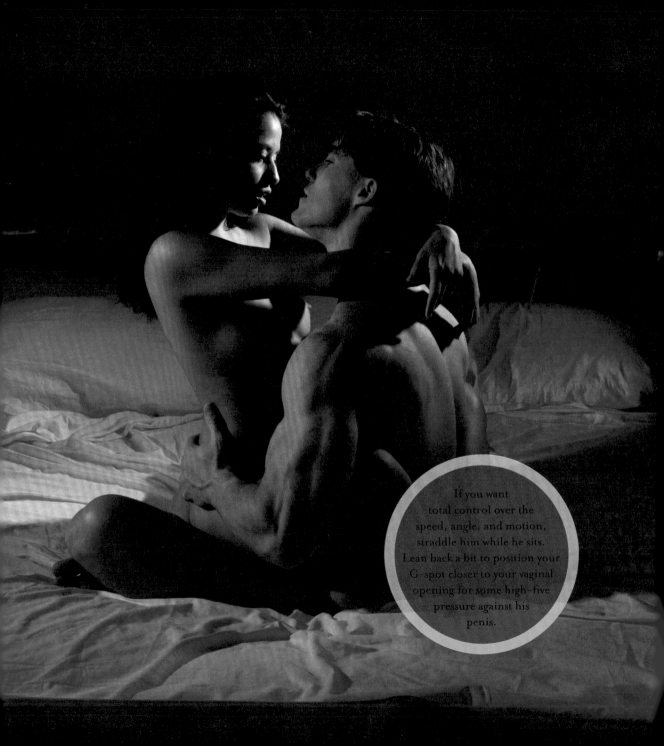

If you want total control over the speed, angle, and motion, straddle him while he sits. Lean back a bit to position your G-spot closer to your vaginal opening for some high-five pressure against his penis.

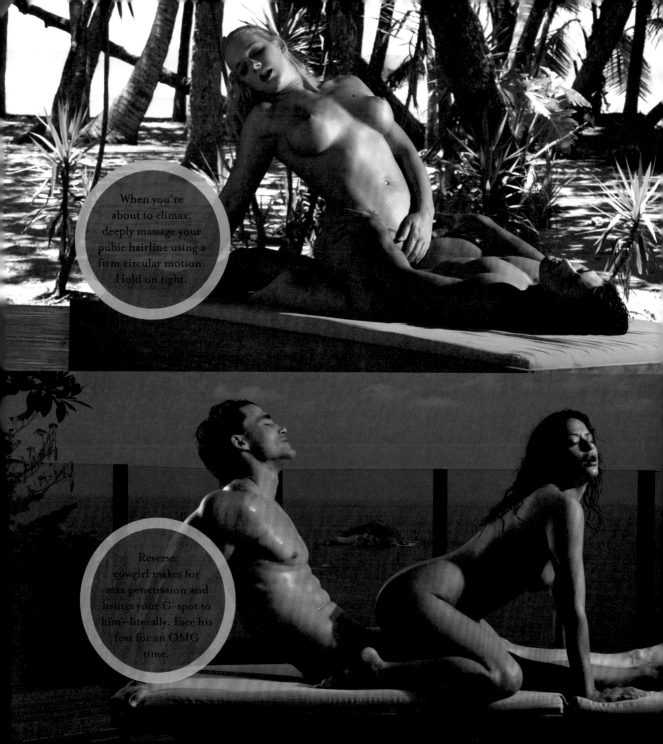

When you're about to climax, deeply massage your pubic hairline using a firm circular motion. Hold on tight.

Reverse cowgirl makes for max penetration and brings your G-spot to him—literally. Face his feet for an OMG time.

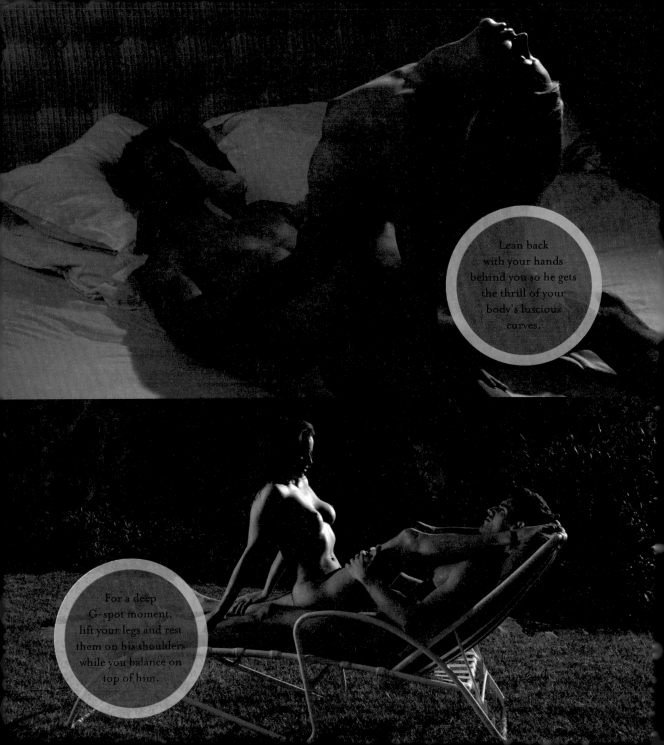

Lean back
with your hands
behind you so he gets
the thrill of your
body's luscious
curves.

For a deep
G-spot moment,
lift your legs and rest
them on his shoulders
while you balance on
top of him.

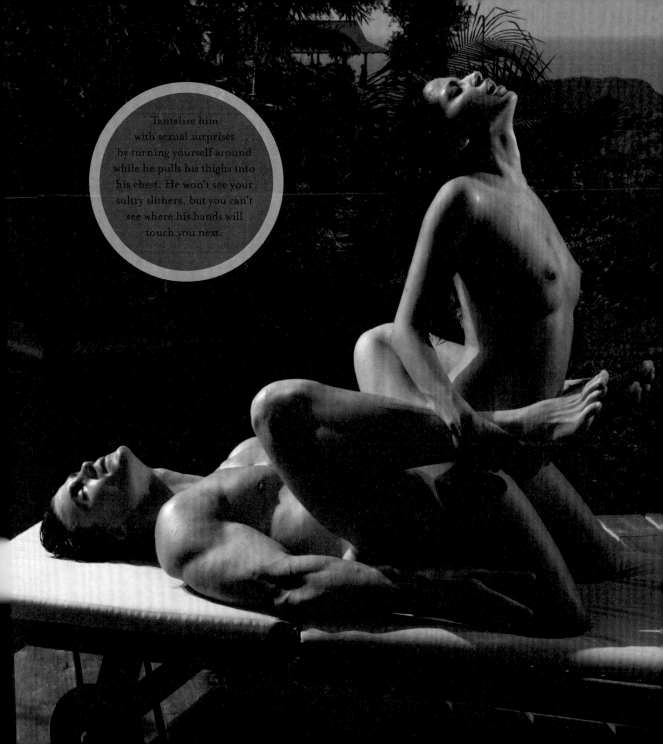

Tantalize him
with sexual surprises
by turning yourself around
while he pulls his thighs into
his chest. He won't see your
sultry slithers, but you can't
see where his hands will
touch you next.

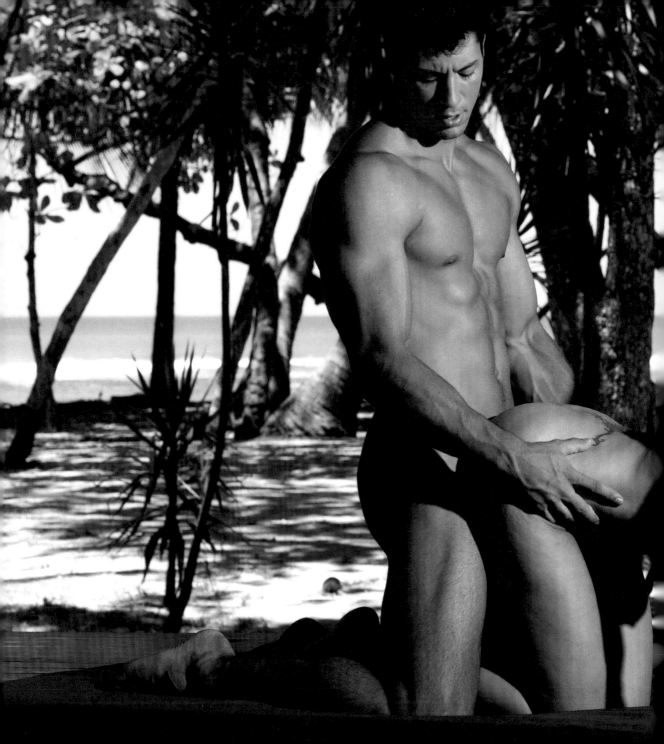

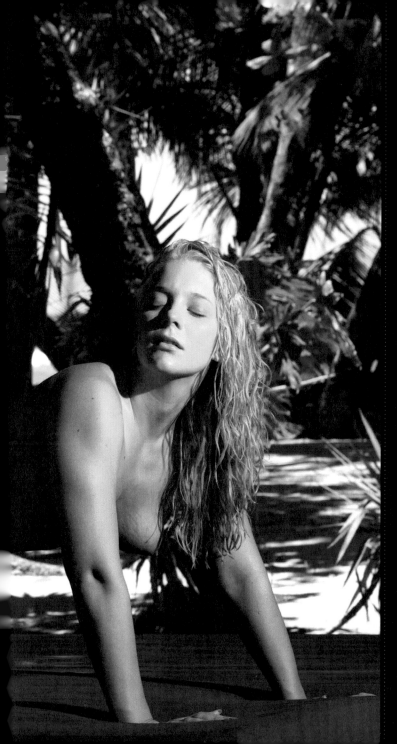

From Behind

Rear entry is a surefire way to hit all your hottest spots. Plus, coming in from behind leaves his hands free to give your bottom some TLC, your breasts a caress, and your love nub all the rub-a-dub-dub it needs.

If you lie flat on your front and open your legs wide, he can kneel between them and inch down until he is lying on top of you so his whole upper body is one with yours, giving ultrasensual head-to-toe connection.

Doing it doggie style will also automatically place him on target to stimulate your cervix, and it's a good move for directing him to your AFE zone because the slant makes him naturally hit the front wall of your vagina. For an extra bonus, rear entry is the position most likely to hit your G-spot.

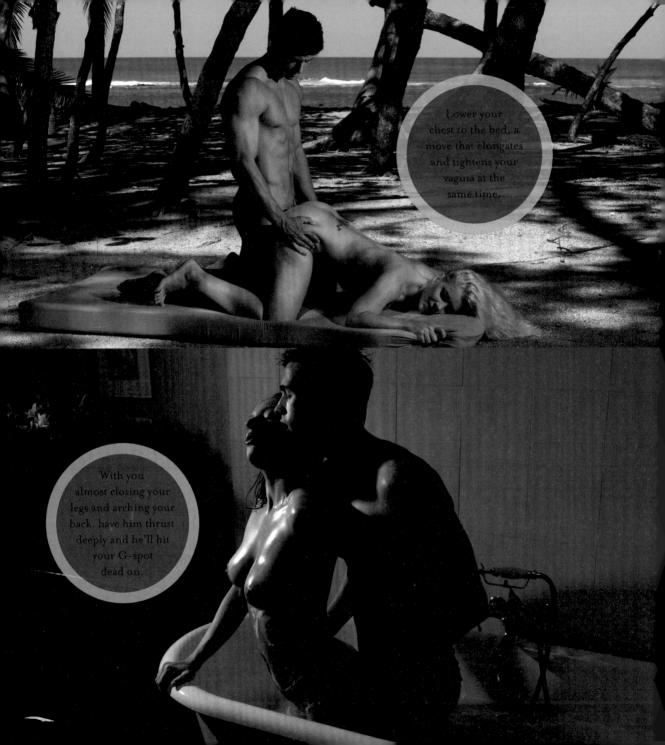

Lower your
chest to the bed, a
move that elongates
and tightens your
vagina at the
same time.

With you
almost closing your
legs and arching your
back, have him thrust
deeply and he'll hit
your G-spot
dead on.

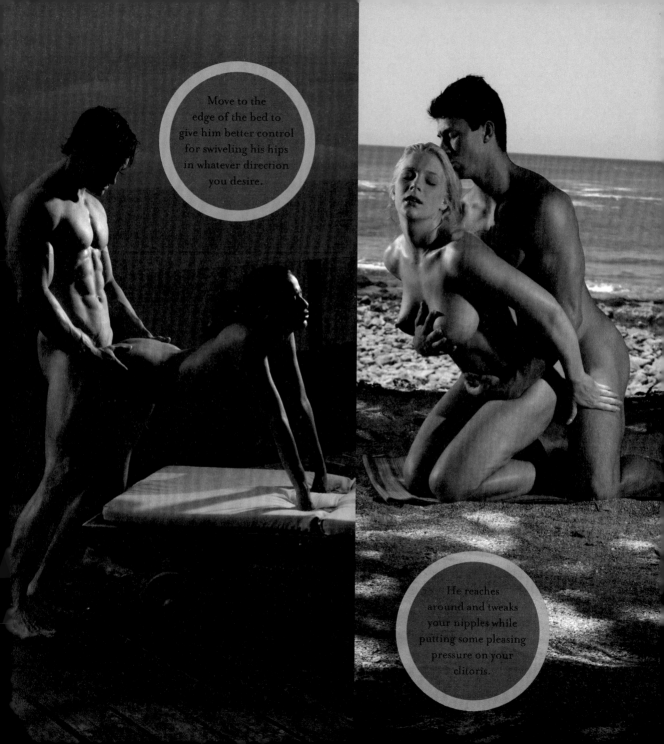

Move to the
edge of the bed to
give him better control
for swiveling his hips
in whatever direction
you desire.

He reaches
around and tweaks
your nipples while
putting some pleasing
pressure on your
clitoris.

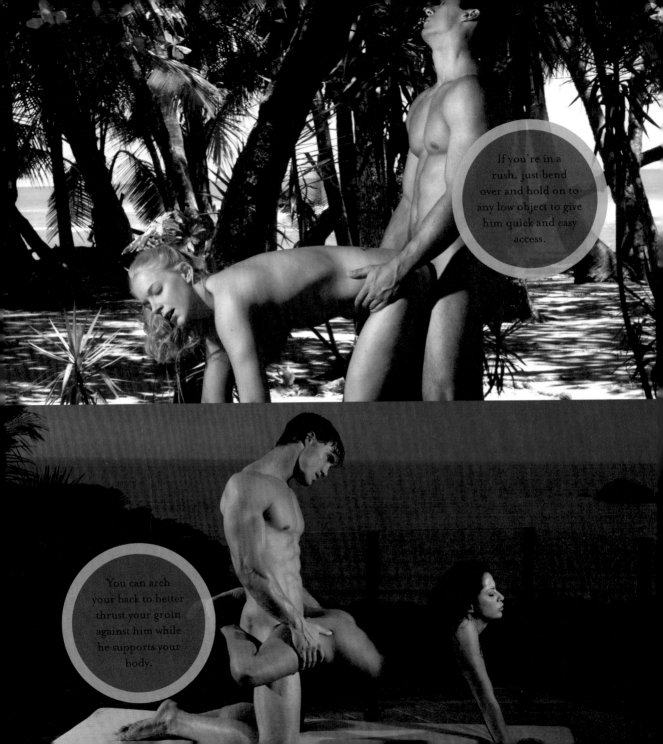

If you're in a rush, just bend over and hold on to any low object to give him quick and easy access.

You can arch your back to better thrust your groin against him while he supports your body.

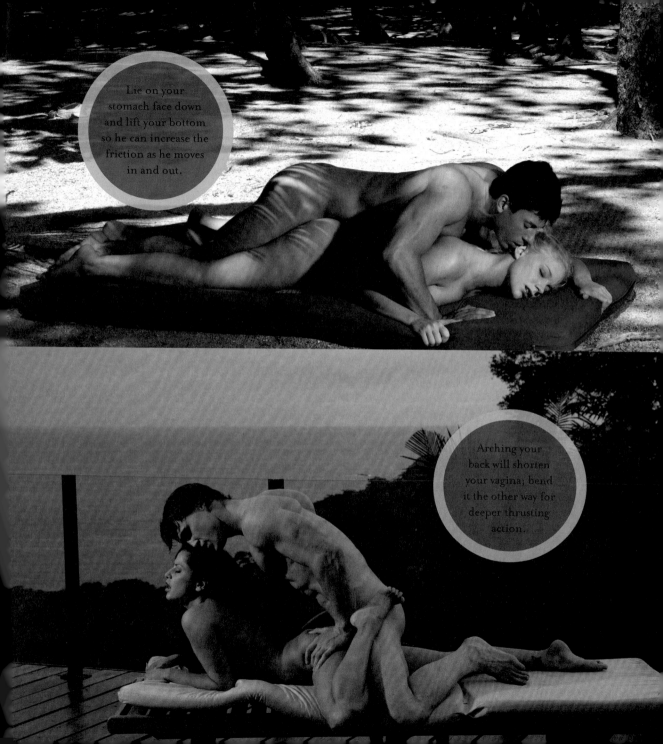

Lie on your
stomach face down
and lift your bottom
so he can increase the
friction as he moves
in and out.

Arching your
back will shorten
your vagina; bend
it the other way for
deeper thrusting
action.

Side to Side

Lie facing each other on your sides, superclose together. Raise your upper leg and help him to slide inside you, then drape the leg over his and tighten around it. This relaxing pose is perfect for slow, sensuous lovemaking. The moves will keep your bodies melded from head to toe. Cuddling on your sides with your legs intertwined and hugging each other close offers the most skin-to-skin contact, while spooning, with him snuggled up to you from behind, will allow him to enter you and intimately hold you oh! so close.

Lie on your back while he lies on his side, turned toward you. Swing both legs over his hips and thighs, making a bridge over them. He then him gently thrusts into you. This is a no-rush, no-stress pose for snuggling. But when you want to climax, it's easy to touch yourself or he can use his top hand to stimulate you.

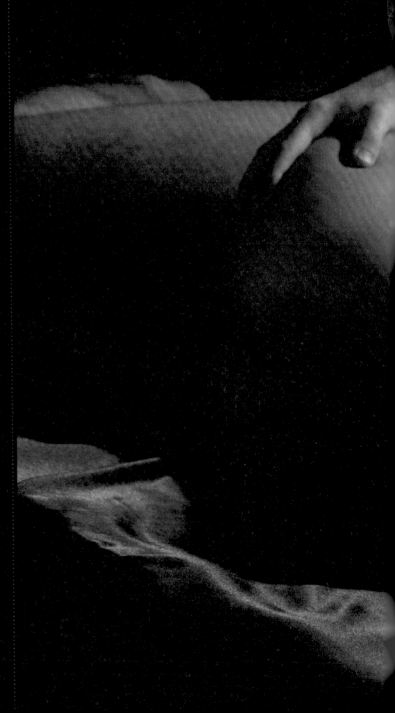

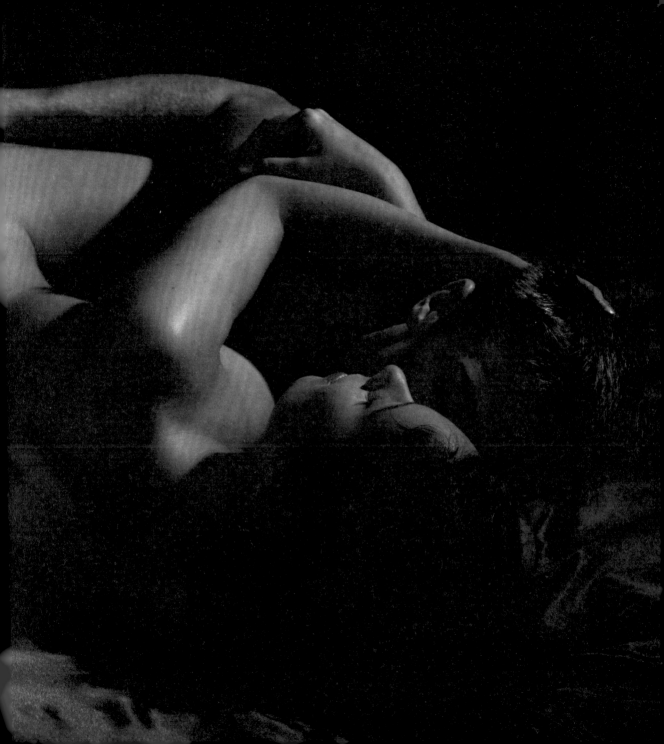

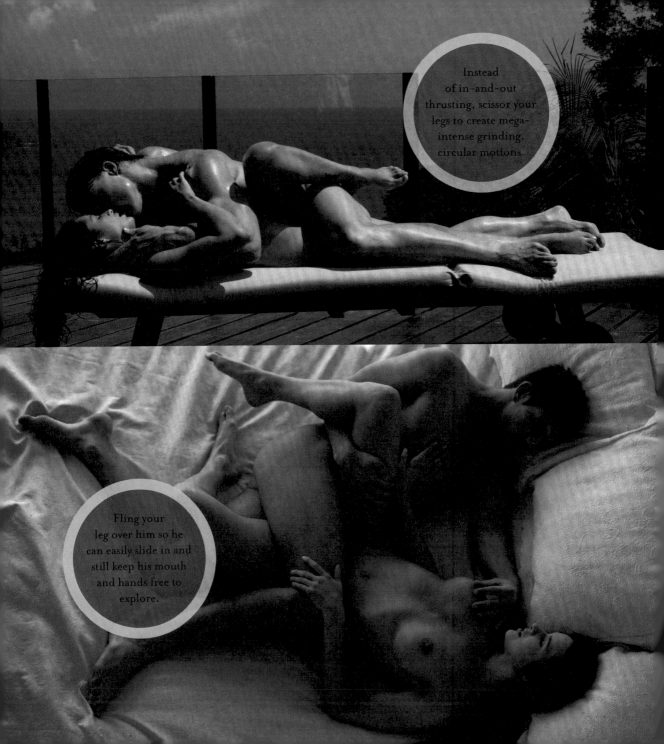

Instead of in-and-out thrusting, scissor your legs to create mega-intense grinding, circular motions.

Fling your leg over him so he can easily slide in and still keep his mouth and hands free to explore.

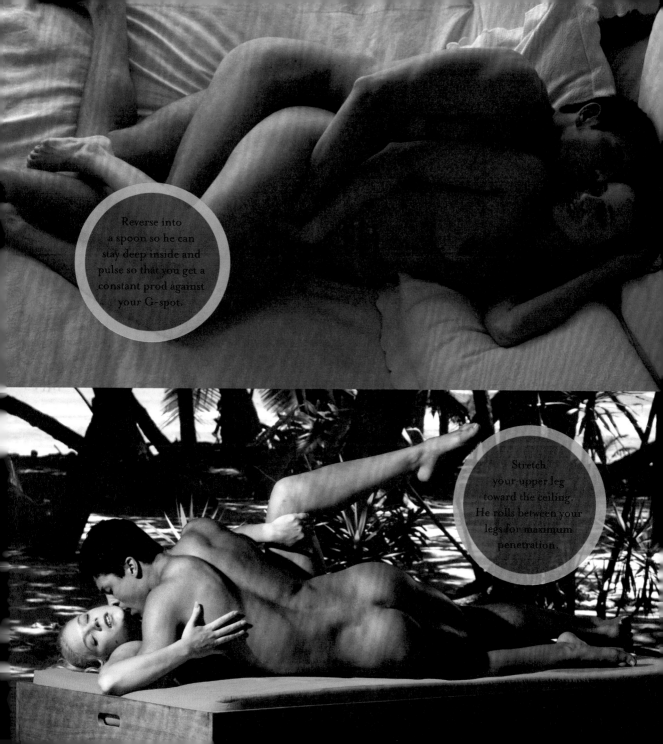

Reverse into a spoon so he can stay deep inside and pulse so that you get a constant prod against your G-spot.

Stretch your upper leg toward the ceiling. He rolls between your legs for maximum penetration.

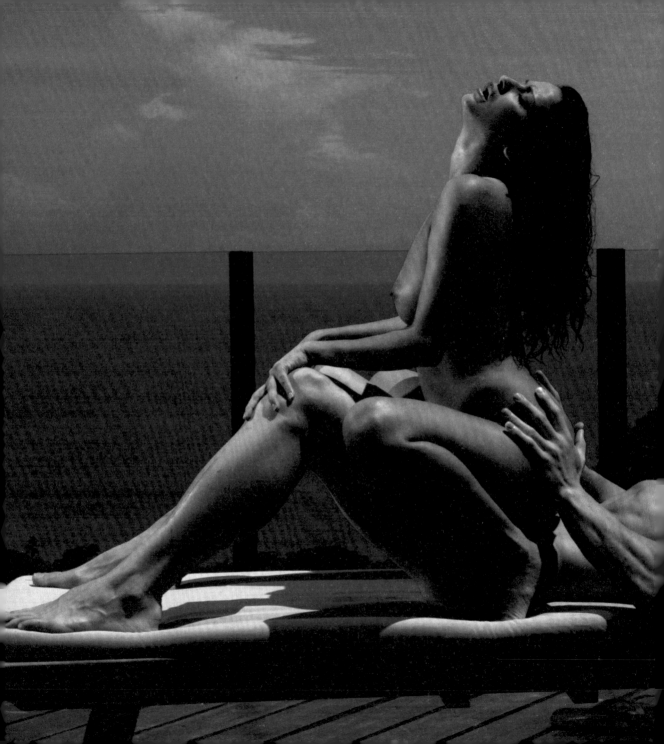

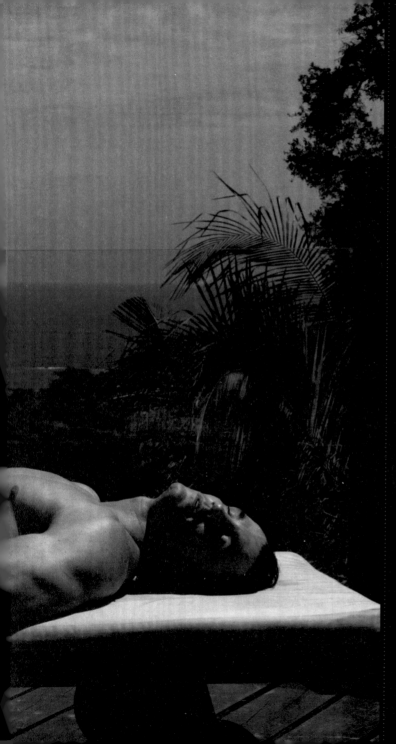

Breathless Bliss

You can actually use your breath to improve your orgasm. Here's how to pant your way to pleasure.

❖ Pick up the pace. The faster you breathe, the more excited you get.

❖ Training the diaphragm, the muscular partition that separates the chest and abdominal cavity, can really increase the intensity of your orgasm. Concentrate on bringing each exhale up from your belly so that you feel your diaphragm contracting to force the air out. During sex, as you feel an orgasm approach, breathe more strongly and consciously than usual, forcing each breath out from the diaphragm. You'll increase the tension through your abdomen and upper body, raising the elation of your ecstasy.

❖ Breathing through the nose is good for de-stressing, but for great sex you need to breathe deeply through your mouth.

Get in Sync

It's a fact of life: When it comes to orgasmic payoff, men speed-race and women meander. This doesn't mean that he always has to drive with the brakes on. These randy romps are designed to keep you both cruising along at the same pleasure pace.

❖ When both of you need a little extra zip, get into missionary and raise your right leg until your knee is even with his left shoulder. (Leave your other leg flat on the bed.) He should refocus his thrusts toward the inner thigh of your raised leg, which keeps things hot for him while creating tighter penetration and more pressure on the clitoris for you.

❖ Give yourselves some slack. Orgasm is really just the release of extreme body tension—the more tension you have, the more pleasurable the release. Most people pick up the pace as they begin to reach their passion peak, but that also has a backfire effect of dulling the senses as your body prepares for its big bang. Slowing your stroke down will increase the tension and result in a more explosive ending.

❖ Mix it up. Resist the urge to thrust fast, hard, and deep in a repetitive one-two pattern. Instead, shuffle slow, deep thrusts with quick, shallow ones. Start with mostly shallow thrusts that target the first third of the vagina—the most sensitive part. Increase the number of deep thrusts, but guide him to go in slowly and come out quickly; the fast withdrawals will generate even more sensation for the clitoris.

❖ Reversing roles will increase his staying power. Tell him to lie still while you do all the heavy lifting and pushing.

❖ Change your position a few times. The momentary lapse can halt your momentum.

❖ When he needs to slow down, have him move his pelvis in a circle or up and down against your love-nub. He'll get a break from high-intensity stimulation, and you'll receive focused attention where it often matters most.

❖ You can get a jump start by having sex even if he isn't fully erect. As long as he is at least as tall as you, have him sit on his raised heels as you squat over him, face to face, with your thighs spread, and guide his penis inside. Then you can take some of the weight off his back by leaning back on one arm while holding on to him with the other.

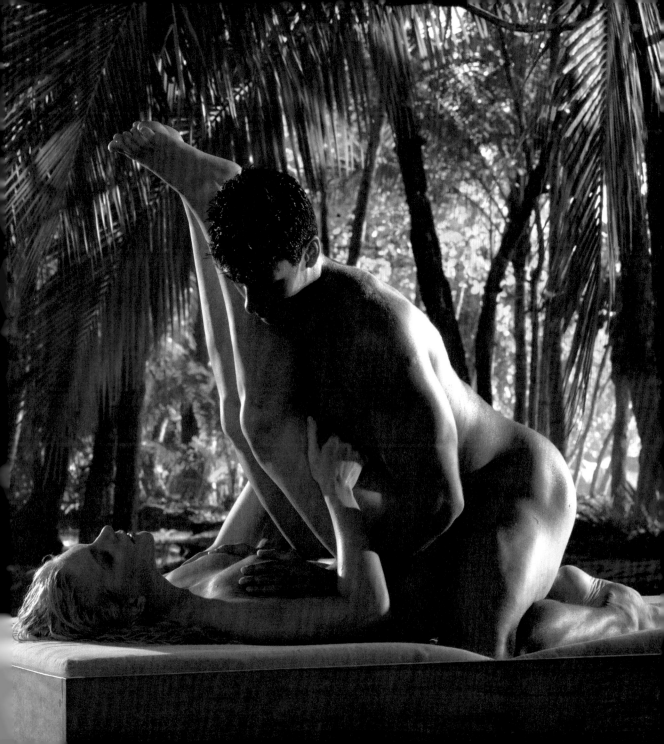

60-Second Climaxes

The moves that work best when you're in a hurry are generally standing up, especially if space is tight. Unfortunately, the male and female physiques rarely match up in a way that makes this feasible. Doing it on the stairs (you one step higher) or on an incline evens things out.

   If you don't have time for foreplay, the best way to get a catch-your-breath orgasm is from the deep penetration that comes from either you-on-top or rear entry.

✤ Anything rear entry will give the deep penetration needed for quick sex and let his penis brush up against all the hot spots situated on the ultrasensitive front of your vaginal wall.

✤ Rear entry and you-on-top are also fabulous for moregasming and multitasking because they leave his hands free to wander. Of course, you can always lend yourself a helping hand as well.

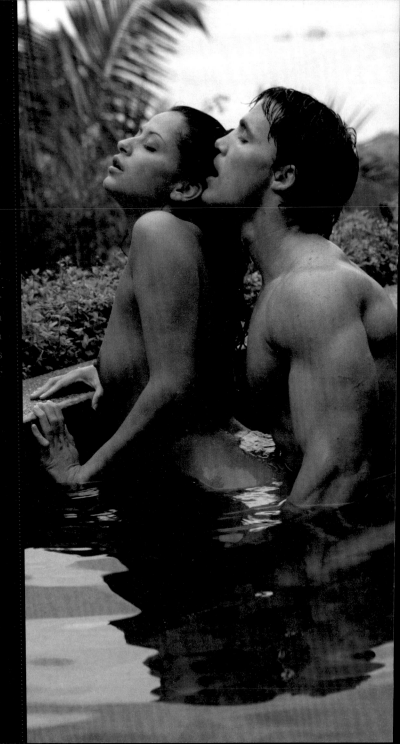

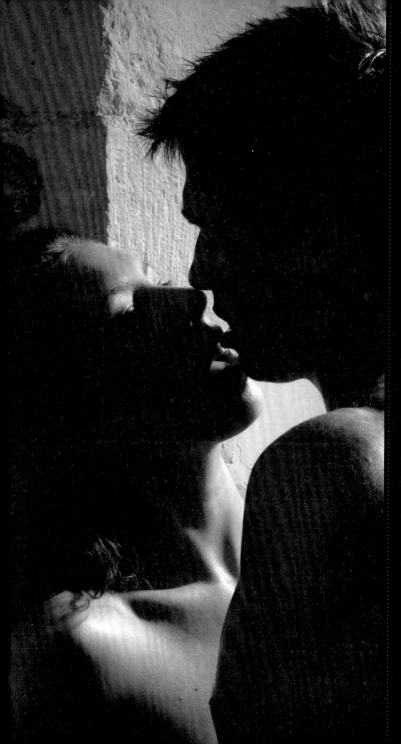

Four handy moves

While making whoopy, don't forget to use your hands to up the pleasure. Here are four tried-and-true tricks.

◈ Drawing you close by grabbing your hips or encircling you with his arms to bring you in tight shows how much he's craving you.

◈ Applying pressure by lightly scratching his nails against your back or gently tugging your hair adds a wild, uncontrolled element.

◈ He can stroke your breasts—they're not just for foreplay.

◈ Cupping your cheeks in his hands and gazing into your eyes creates an intense connection that goes beyond saying, "I love you."

Under Pressure

Work your muscles to pump up the pleasure. First, flex. Buffing up your pelvic muscles will give you bigger, more intense, and just plain more orgasms without even leaving your bed. To get started, practice squeezing the same muscles you use to control your urine flow. (If you're not sure which these are, try stopping mid-stream next time you pee—bingo!) Work up to 15 reps of squeezing, twice a day, holding for five seconds and releasing.

Once you're in control, go for the burn during sex.

✤ When he's thrusting in and out, squeeze really tightly each time before he re-enters.

✤ Sit on top of him and, without thrusting, squeeze powerfully ten times.

✤ Do it from behind—once he's inside, begin contracting your muscles. You'll press his penis against the front wall of your vagina, where your G-spot lives.

✤ Squeeze when he's about to come.

✤ Give the ultrasensitive head of his penis a massage by clamping down just as he enters you. He'll have to squeeze in, creating fabulous friction.

✤ Milk him like you're a dairy farmer—when he's inside of you, tighten and push out, then squeeze in a constricting manner, but without pulling him all the way back in. Push out, constrict, pull in a little, and push out and constrict again until he explodes.

✤ When you're on the bottom, clench. You'll lift your pelvis a couple of inches off the bed and increase blood flow to your pelvic area to make orgasm easier.

✤ For a red-hot orgasm, squat on your partner, facing him, while he sits up. Thrust toward each other ten times. Stop and squeeze powerfully with your pelvic muscles ten times.

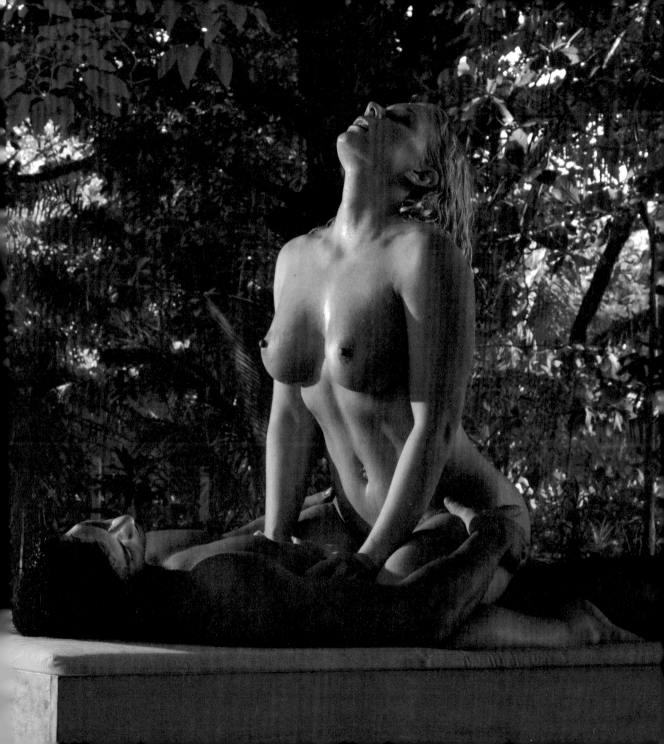

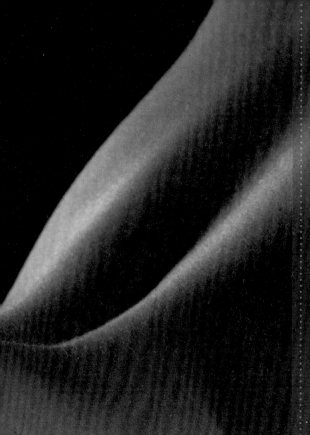

6: ADVANCED TECHNIQUES

After you've mastered the ways to make your whole body feel oh! so delicious, take it to the next level with these not-for-beginners moves. Even the nicest of nice girls can tire of the same old same old, so now's the time to challenge yourself with some exciting, never-felt-before thrill.

From raising the pleasure quotient with everything from high-tech sex toys and around-the-house props to anal exploration and multiorgasmic techniques, there's a whole well of blood-pumping pleasure just waiting to be tapped.

Bottom's Up

Your bottom is too often sidelined during sex. Big mistake. The anus is packed with love-happy nerve endings, but anal sex is one of the truly advanced ways to get carnal, and necessary precautions should be taken. Here are a few ins-and-outs of making you swoon for booty calls.

Re-lax-ation The key to making a full-bottom bungee jump land smoothly is to be fully relaxed. Start off with a long, warm bath, or better yet, be on the receiving end of a few electrifying orgasms first.

Start clean Always a good idea with any sex act, this is particularly smart for backdoor action. Making sure you're well washed should be fine, but if you're really concerned about cleanliness, try douching your anus in the shower before coming to the bedroom.

Lubricate This cannot be overemphasized. The bottom does not secrete fluid, so grease up. Silicone lubes (versus glycerine ones) are slippery and stay that way. Whatever kind of lube you choose, use liberally.

Take the slow lane Have him test the waters before letting his johnny jump in. Starting with one, then two (well-lubed) fingers, he should gently stroke the region right around the opening—gently pushing at the center—but not actually penetrating, so then he can just inch his finger or tongue in for a quick skinny-dip.

Stay shallow You don't have to go for a deep plunge. The highest concentration of nerve endings is around the anal opening itself.

Hot-diggedy-dogged The best position is rear entry. After you arrange yourselves, he can rub his penis against your opening, which should relax the anus. As the sphincter muscles periodically contract, the anus appears to "wink," which is his signal to slide in.

Get in shape The rectum is not a straight tube; it's more like an S. So when he goes in, he should adjust his angle and aim for your belly button. If it starts to hurt after a few inches, he's probably hit the curve. Have him stop and pull back a smidge to let your bottom adjust. The more you relax, the more your rectum elongates. After a moment, he can go a little deeper, aiming toward your head.

Finish clean Anal bacteria from waste products (poop) can remain on the penis even if you use a condom, so don't switch from anal to vaginal or oral sex before thoroughly washing anything, including fingers, that enter your bottom.

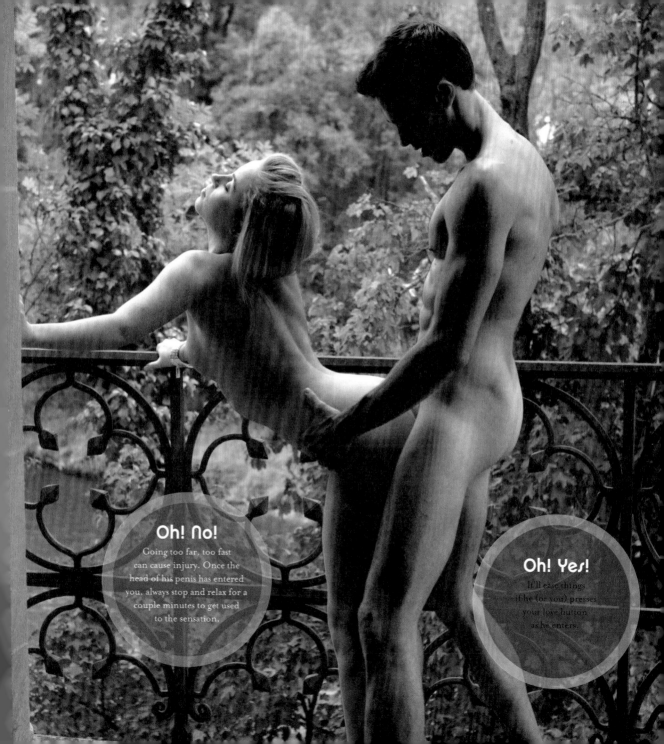

Oh! No!

Going too far, too fast can cause injury. Once the head of his penis has entered you, always stop and relax for a couple minutes to get used to the sensation.

Oh! Yes!

It'll ease things if he (or you) presses your love button as he enters.

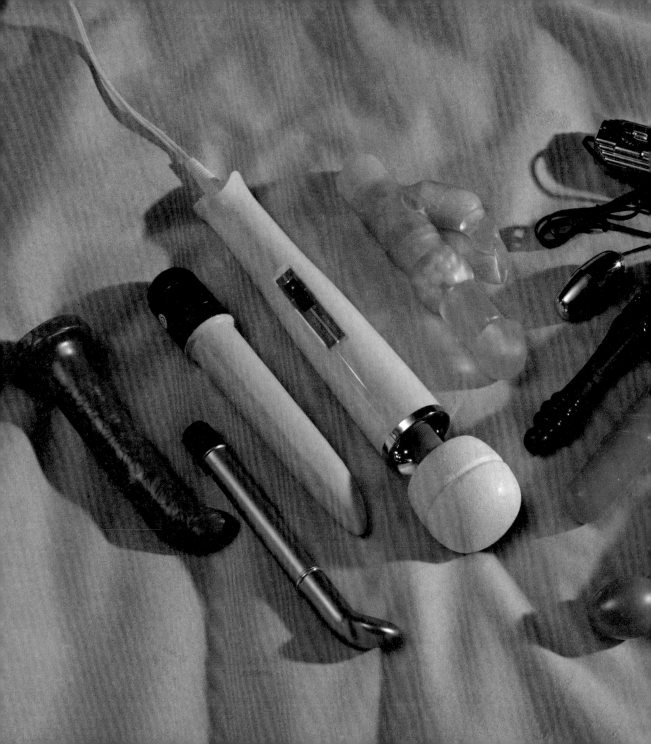

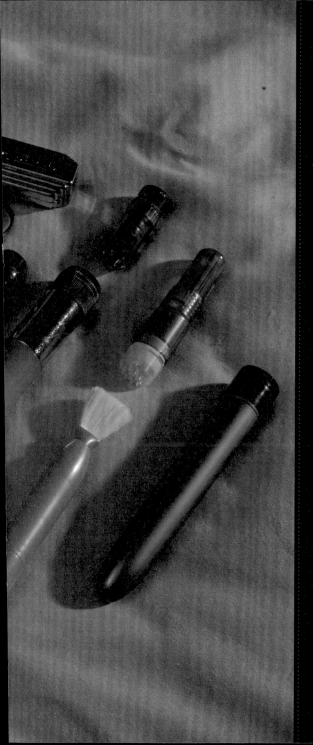

Toy Story

Here's what sex toys can do for you: give you body-boggling orgasms, give him body-boggling orgasms, give you both body-boggling orgasms.

Here's what sex toys will not do for you: make you feel weird or make you so addicted to using your new gadget that you won't be able to come any other way or take out your garbage.

Using sex toys makes you a better lover simply because anything that keys you into your own arousal gives you clues to bring into your bedtime play.

There is a huge array of discreet, fun, easy-to-use doo-dahs available—with or without a partner. Toys seem to come in so many different shapes, sizes, colors, materials, and speeds that a girl could have a different model for every day of the year (including leap year).

Size matters If you want a tool with measure-ments he can only fantasize having, look for anything with words for magnitude in the name, such as "colossal" or "titan." Just make sure you pay attention to the dimensions of these toys, as some of these giants can be the size of a rolling pin! Since good things also come in small packages, opt for an item that says "mini" or "pocket" if you prefer something portable and easy to maneuver.

Orgasms on demand Practically any vibrator will do, but for a high-tech thrill, try a hands-free strap-on vibrator that's powered remotely. After slipping on the G-string or panty, wait for your partner to tantalize you via the control. (Just don't lose it!)

Outer enlightenment Small and compact, these clitoral vibrators don't have fancy shafts topped with gizmos or gadgets. What they do have is a head, a ball, a bullet, or an egg designed to stimulate the clitoris; many are controlled by a small remote attached to a thin wire. Few look like what they really are. Some are even shaped like dolphins, bunnies, or mutant human megatongues. No matter which design you choose, the basic operation is the same—focused vibrations at varying speeds and intensities.

Inner enlightenment Innies such as wands and dildos are designed to work like a penis and to be thrust into the vagina, sometimes with the added ooh-la-la of vibration, rotation, or some other kind of internal humdinger. Many have curved tips or knobbed sides to give your G-spot a friendly how-de-do.

Every which way If you can't decide, or want it all (and why not?), dual-action vibrators come with a rotating or vibrating dildo as well as a clitoral stimulator (often a twirling shaft for vaginal penetration plus a clit stimulator) for the best of both worlds.

Give him a boost A cock ring will make him last longer, stay harder, and heighten the intensity and length of his orgasm. A vibrating cock ring will make you want him to last forever.

Get bum rushed Slip in a strand of heavily lubed anal beads and pull them out very slowly just as you climax. Or try a small butt plug. If you really love a backdoor bounce, opt for the vibrating kind.

Preen your breasts Adorn them with clip-on nipple rings. If you prefer more pressure, there are clamps—vibrating or no-frills—that lightly pinch the nipples.

Take a little walk on the wild side Try a beginner kink set. Most come with fuzzy handcuffs, a blindfold or mask, a soft paddle, nipple clamps, a mini vibrator, and a scented candle for wax play.

Make your sex life even juicier Steady clitoral contact is your ticket to ride. But without adequate lubrication, it can become a rocky journey. Packing on some grease allows your hot zones to be directly, continually stroked without causing painful friction. Make sure the kind of lube you choose is compatible with your birth control and your other sex toys. The hands-down favorite for couples is his-and-hers lubes that cool him down and heat her up. Flavored gels also get the tongues-up.

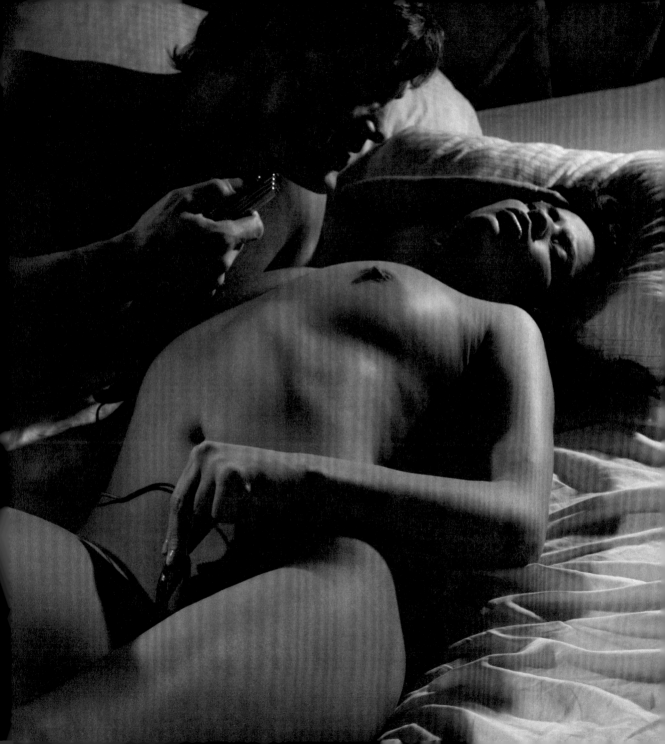

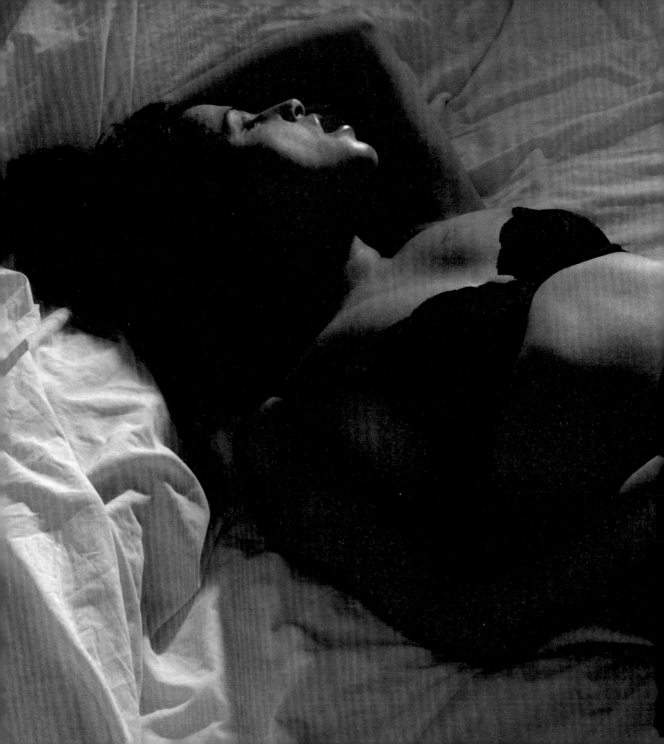

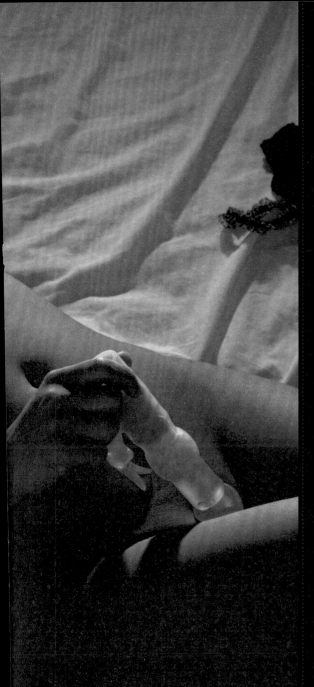

Operating Instructions

You have your new toy in hand. Now what?

Since some vibrators and dildos look more like a child's toy than something purchased to put on your body's most intimate parts, and they often come without directions, here are some quick tips and techniques to help you get started.

❖ Send feel-good tremors through both of you—place a bullet-shaped buzz buddy at the base of his penis when you're on top and grind against it.

❖ To blast orgasm during missionary, slip a small vibrator over your clitoris while he's on top. His heart will go pitter-patter over the extra pulse on his nerve endings.

❖ At around 2,000 cycles per minute, the purr from a vibrator can sometimes be too intense. One way to take it down a notch without losing any of the pleasure is to place a washcloth over your genitals.

❖ Try doing it doggie style and have him doubly stimulate you by gently rubbing the vibrator across your love bump as he enters you.

❖ Don't limit yourself to the major erogenous zones. The entire body is chock-full of tingling nerves just waiting to be given a caress. The thinner the skin in the area you're touching, the more responsive it will be. Try rubbing your toy along your neck,

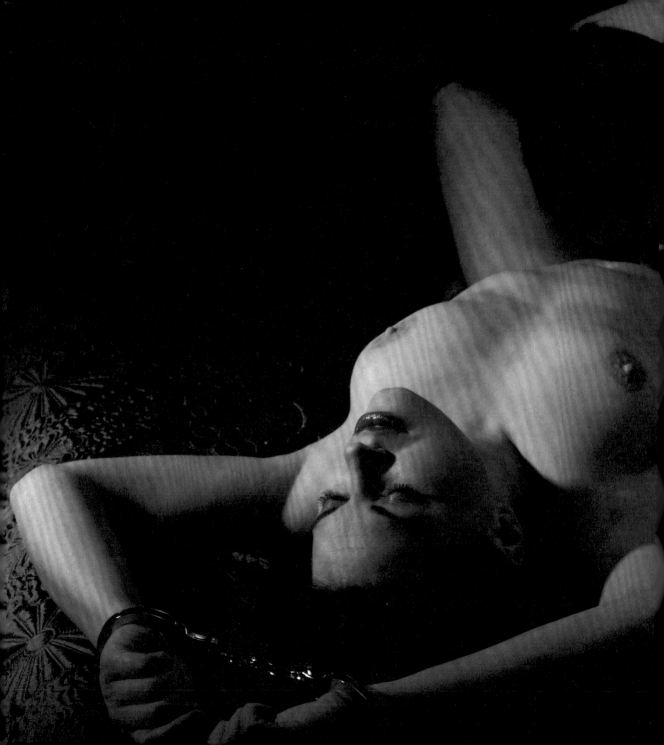

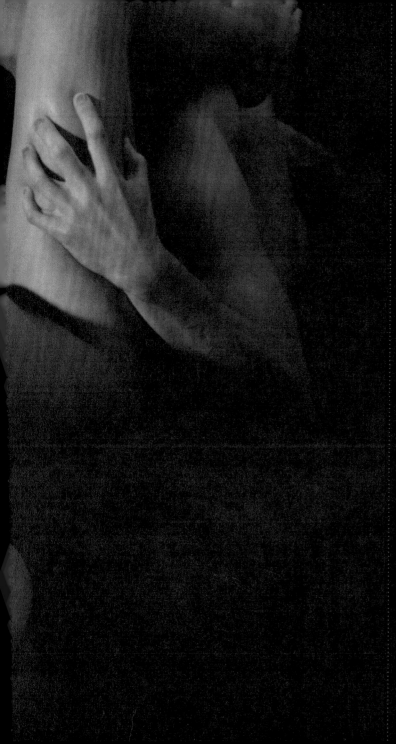

tummy, inner thighs, inner forearms, and temples for some out-of-this-world sensations.

✤ Some women find direct clitoral stimulation too intense, so work your vibrator around the bump.

✤ If you have a G-spot vibrator, experiment with twisting it around in your vagina to hit all the different inner spots.

✤ Don't limit yourself to one stroke when there's an entire world of battery-operated moves out there for you to enjoy. Try going in a circular motion, back and forth, switching between thrusting deep and shallow in-and-outs—play around until you find a few motions that wow you.

✤ If you have a penetrative vibe or dildo, wiggle it around in your vagina, trying different depths. Hold it just at the opening of the vagina. If there's a larger head at the tip of the vibrator, try very shallow dips with just the tip.

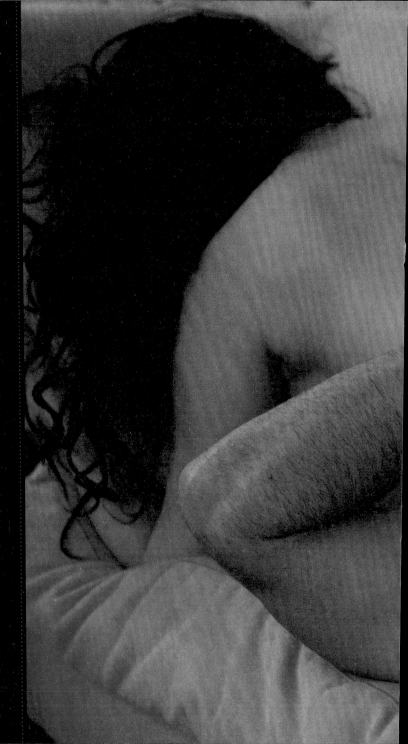

✧ Work your plaything everywhere else—rubbing your anus, stroking his penis, squeezing your nipples, pressing against your vaginal lips, probing his testicles.

✧ Have him bring in a stunt double and use his tongue on your love knob as he slowly inserts your sex toy deep inside you.

✧ Lie on your belly with a pillow positioned under your hips so you can buzz your vibrator to stimulate your vagina and clitoris from behind.

✧ Putting the vibe on your genitals, squeeze your thighs and butt cheeks together, then release. Repeat until you detonate.

✧ For increased sensation for both of you, apply a warming lube designed for sex to his penis right before he enters you. Keep it dollop-sized or it will make your action too slippery.

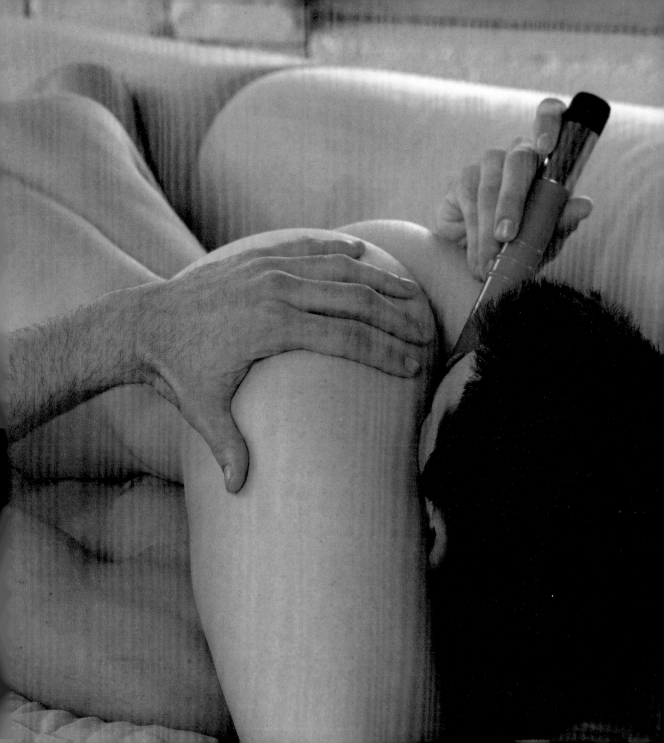

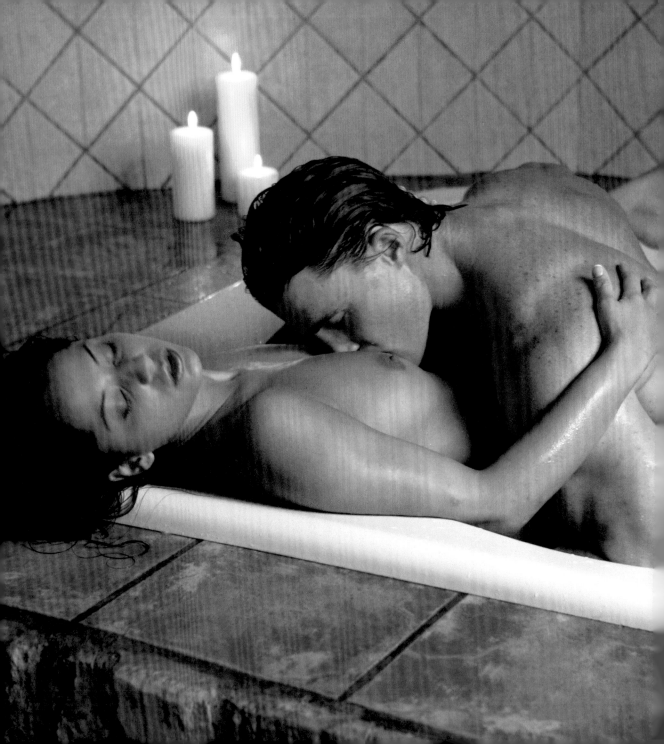

House Raid

Make like MacGyver and turn everyday objects into your own personalized sex toy chest.

Go electric   Buy an electric toothbrush (or a new attachment—and make sure you reserve it just for play). Cover the bristles with a small soft cloth, turn it on, and gently run it against yourself.

Turn down the volume   Cell phones make great sex toys. Skip the lascivious texts and set yours to vibrate for an instant ring-a-ling.

Raid the costume box   Dressing up is a cheap way to play out your favorite Star Wars or action-hero fantasy.

Do the laundry   Making love on the washing machine during the spin cycle will feel like a giant vibrator.

Try a homemade sling   Get in rear-entry position and wrap a towel or a strong, wide belt under your hips. He can pull both ends to lift your hips and butt higher and control your motions as he thrusts in and out.

Get decorated   Take a beaded necklace (one without exposed string or wire), lube it up, then wrap it around his penis and roll it up and down.

Bounce on an exercise ball   Roll it out and arch back with your legs spread and feet flat on the ground. He can either kneel in front of you or balance over you in push-up position. The constant motion of the ball will hit new places inside with every roll.

Bend over the sofa   Have him sit on the back of the sofa to brace himself for your mounting. Swing your leg across to the front to pull your hips back and forth as you rock yourself to ecstasy.

Balance on a chair   Swivel chairs are perfect for custom-tinkering with his angle. Just sit and have him kneel on a pillow in front of you. For stable chairs, make like an aerialist and, facing the chair, balance your arms on the seat. He can hold your hips high and inch his way in. You'll feel like you're floating.

Groove on a beanbag   It's a lot like making love in water—it supports you and holds your bodies in ways you're not usually slanted, so everyday positions take on a whole new dimension.

Grab the headboard   The right angle means you can sit up and draw your legs up high and wide, giving him direct aim at your inner hot

Moregasms

If you believe that you can never have too much of a good thing—particularly when it comes to sex—here's some good news: Women's bodies are styled to create unlimited pleasure. The beauty of the clitoris is that it doesn't need any R & R after you climax. As long as it gets stimulation, you'll keep coming, so you can have as many repeat performances of bliss as you desire.

There's more than one way to multiply your orgasms.

- Take your time frolicking with foreplay. Orgasm, don't orgasm—it doesn't matter. The more stimulation you get, the more primed your body gets, making it easier to move on to multiple peaks.

- Putting your pleasure on delay puts you on the fast track for a series of sweet spasms. Holding off from going woo-hoo for as long as possible builds up the sexual tension to triple-degree temperatures. Your body gets into a state of high sexpectation so even after your first explosive orgasm you're ready for more.

- Don't stop. If your usual passion schedule is get caressed, get carnal, and then conk out in a postcoital coma, reprogram yourself to retrace your steps back to foreplay after you climax. Your body is already sparking, so it won't take long for the bonfire to begin.

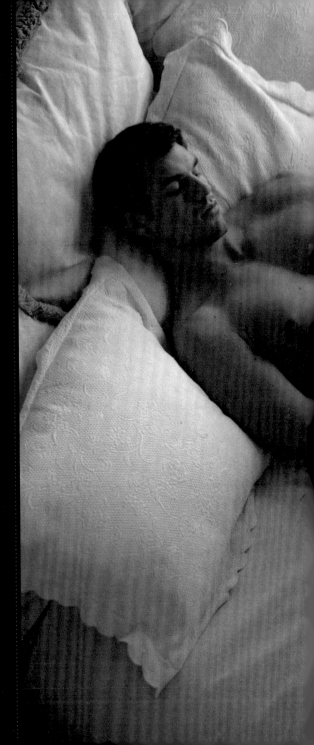

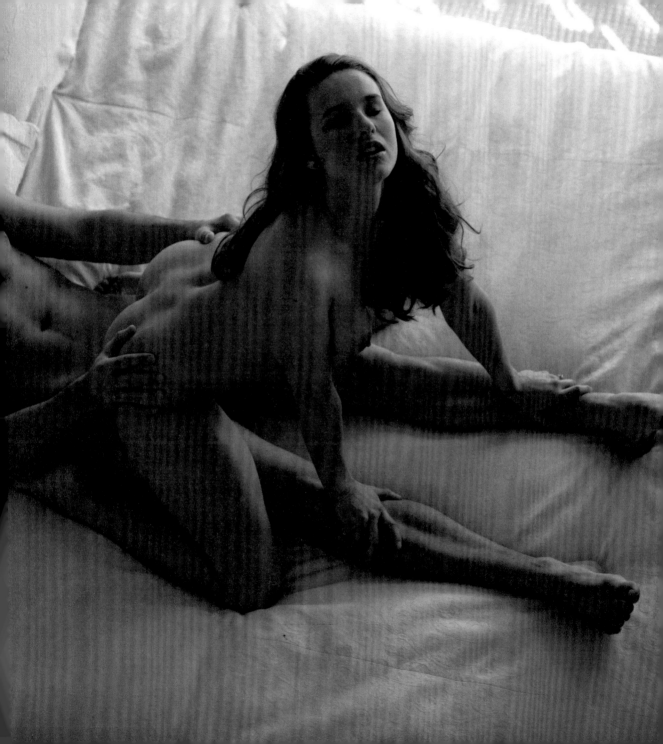

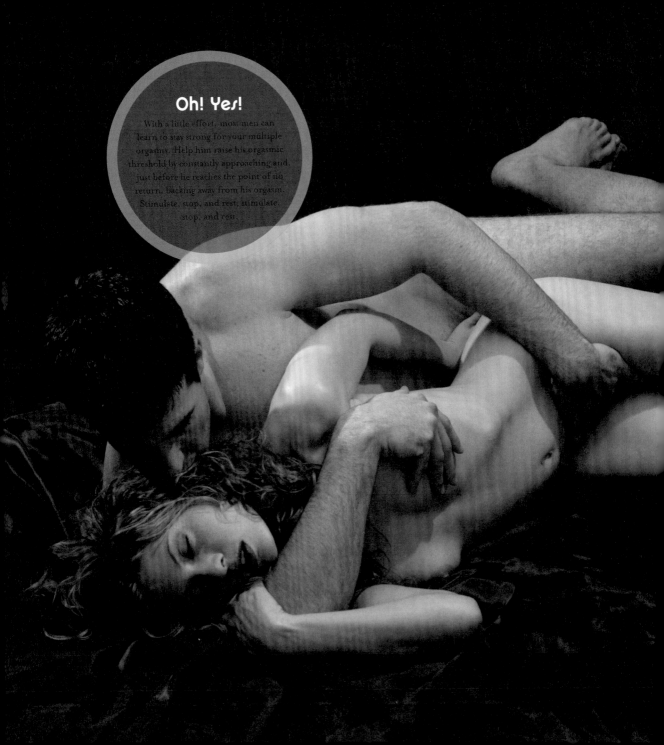

Oh! Yes!

With a little effort, most men can learn to stay strong for your multiple orgasms. Help him raise his orgasmic threshold by constantly approaching and, just before he reaches the point of no return, backing away from his orgasm. Stimulate, stop, and rest; stimulate, stop, and rest.

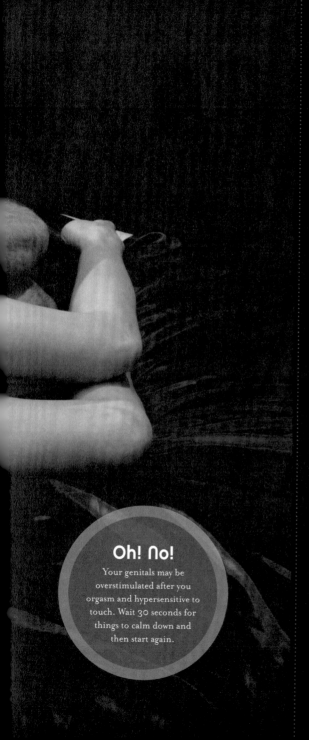

Oh! No!

Your genitals may be overstimulated after you orgasm and hypersensitive to touch. Wait 30 seconds for things to calm down and then start again.

◈ Get out of your rut. The more different kinds of stimulation you experience, the easier it is to leapfrog from pleasure wave to pleasure wave. So, once you've climaxed, simply switch to caressing another body part or change your lovemaking position.

◈ If you need something more to send you over the edge, contract your pelvic muscles while your partner alternates between stroking the inside of your vagina and your clitoris. Continue until you bliss out on a crescendo of orgasms.

◈ Don't wait to exhale. Most people tend to hold their breath when they hit their peak. But continuing to push breath through your body keeps blood pumping to the genitals rather than being diverted to the rest of your body. If you can, make your breaths slow and long, from the pit of your belly. This sort of deep breathing puts the focus back on your body and all the delicious sensations it's experiencing.

◈ The more stimulation you can get at the crucial moment, the better. Your clitoris is the star, and the best positions are rear entry or sitting backward on him, because they get right to the clitoral point. But if intercourse isn't giving your love nub all the fizzy focus it needs, throw in some hand moves, a vibrator, or some pelvic muscle clenches. Or just send his mouth south. Hitting your G-spot will also do the trick.

The One-Hour Orgasm

Five quick ways to make your carnal connection last from here to eternity.

❖ Take a minute to do what you'd normally do in two seconds. Cranking the action down a few notches makes you acutely aware of every sensation and slows your response rate down in a good way.

❖ Leaning away from each other is perfect for beginning a lovemaking marathon. Sit on top of your partner, facing him. Now fall back in opposite directions with your weight on your elbows or hands or lie flat on your back (whatever makes you happy). He can gently thrust from below for as long as your hearts desire (or his penis holds out—whichever comes first).

❖ A simple sex surrogate technique called "vaginal containment" makes his erection—and your pleasure—last forever. Straddle him or lie on top, with his penis inside you. He shouldn't move at all; he just concentrates on enjoying the sensation of containment without the extra rush of friction.

❖ Hit the right nerves, and sexual euphoria can reach new stratospheres. The two genital nerves that surround the pelvic floor muscles give two kinds of erotic sensation. The first is a sharp twinge that occurs when the clitoris or base of the penis is erect and caressed; the second is a warm, melting feeling that happens when the inside of the vagina or the shaft of the penis is stimulated to climactic heights. Experience both types, one after the other, in a single lovefest, and you'll have what's called a blended orgasm, which can last as long as an hour. One way is to stimulate one part of body—like the clitoris—until it feels too sensitive, then move to the interior of the vagina until it feels aroused, then return to the clitoris and so on and—sigh—on…

❖ Tease yourself. Too many women try to experience an orgasm as quickly as possible. Instead, try prolonging your pleasure by hovering at the brink of orgasm for as long as possible by building up your arousal and then getting your partner to shift his loving attention to a less stimulating part of your body for a few minutes. The beauty of this roller-coaster method is that arousal mounts to such intensity that when you finally let yourself go, you're practically guaranteed an outrageous orgasm.

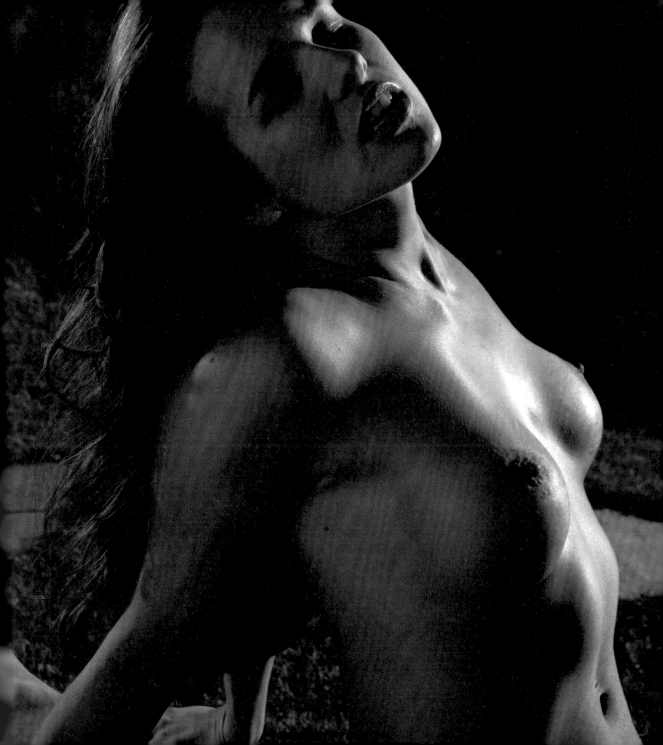

Other Amorata Press Titles

101 Sex Positions: Steamy New Positions from Mild to Wild
Samantha Taylor, $17.95
This sensually illustrated book guides lovers from the straightforward to the adventurous, from the bed to the table, and from "Who's on top?" to who's kneeling, standing, crouching, and holding which limb where.

365 Sex Positions: A New Way Every Day for a Steamy, Erotic Year
Lisa Sweet, $17. 95
From January 1 to December 31, *365 Sex Positions* offers couples an exciting new way to spice up their sex lives every day of the year. With a belief that nothing heats up a couple's bedroom as fast as a new position, this is the ultimate tool for achieving higher levels of pleasure.

Going Down: An Illustrated Guide to Giving Him the Best Blow Job of His Life
Nicci Talbot, $16.95
A perfectly executed blow job will add new thrills to your sex life, strength to your relationship, and leave him weak in the knees—begging for more. Revealing secret tricks and amazing techniques, this book will make you the skilled lover of his dreams.

Orgasms: A Sensual Guide to Female Ecstasy
Nicci Talbot, $16.95
Straight-talking and informative, this book is a girl's best friend when it comes to understanding the physical, psychological, and spiritual factors contributing to great sex and intense orgasms.

Wild and Sexy: The Stunning Book of Thrilling Sex Positions
Laura Leu, $14.95
This book offers the best, boldest, and bravest, including erotic variations on the missionary, doggie, and cowgirl positions; modern examples of Kama Sutra classics; and acrobatic positions for advanced lovemaking.

To order these books call 800-377-2542 or 510-601-8301, fax 510-601-8307, e-mail ulysses@ulyssespress. com, or write to Amorata Press, P.O. Box 3440, Berkeley, CA 94703. All retail orders are shipped free of charge. California residents must include sales tax. Allow two to three weeks for delivery.

About the Author

Lisa Sweet is the author of numerous sexual instruction books, including *365 Sex Positions*, and has had her writing published in newspapers and magazines in the United States, the United Kingdom, France, and Australia.